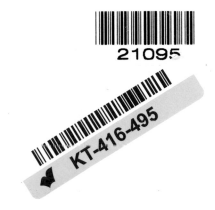

21095

KT-416-495

CHURCHILL'S
Medicolegal
Pocketbook

Commissioning Editor: Timothy Horne
Project Development Manager: Barbara Simmons
Project Manager: Nancy Arnott
Designer: Erik Bigland

CHURCHILL'S
Medicolegal
Pocketbook

Vanessa Machin

MBBS BSc (Hons) AKC FRCS FFAEM DipFMSA
Forensic Medical Examiner for the Metropolitan Police Service

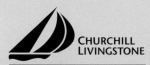

CHURCHILL
LIVINGSTONE

EDINBURGH LONDON NEW YORK PHILADELPHIA
ST LOUIS SYDNEY TORONTO 2003

CHURCHILL LIVINGSTONE
An imprint of Elsevier Science Limited

First published 2003

ISBN 0443 071330

British Library Cataloguing in Publication Data
A catalogue record for this book is available from the British Library

Library of Congress Cataloging in Publication Data
A catalog record for this book is available from the Library of Congress

Note
Medical knowledge is constantly changing. As new information becomes available,
changes in treatment, procedures, equipment and the use of drugs become necessary.
The author and the publishers have taken care to ensure that the information given in
this text is accurate and up to date. However, readers are strongly advised to confirm
that the information, especially with regard to drug usage, complies with the latest
legislation and standards of practice.

 your source for books,
journals and multimedia
in the health sciences
www.elsevierhealth.com

The
publisher's
policy is to use
**paper manufactured
from sustainable forests**

Printed in China

Preface

Despite the fact that they are frequently faced with difficult decisions, healthcare professionals probably feel most insecure when dealing with medicolegal matters. These range from a witness summons to appear in court through the 14-year-old girl who has taken a potentially fatal overdose but is refusing treatment to being asked for help with an Advance Directive. What can you do with a baby who appears to have suffered a non-accidental injury but whose parents are insisting on leaving the Accident and Emergency department? What are the ethical and legal issues if a patient asks you to help them die? How do you deal with a complaint against you?

There are many weighty tomes that cover the legal aspects of the field of medicine. They provide a fascinating insight into the background and derivation of current statute and case law but they are frequently aimed at lawyers rather than healthcare professionals and the latter often find them unpalatable. There are also several specialist books that deal with particular areas such as forensic medicine but there are very few short, practical guides to dealing with most of the medicolegal problems commonly encountered in clinical practice. There is a need for such a handbook as the number of complaints continues to rise, as do the costs of litigation. Recent publicity, such as the Shipman case, has led to calls for changes in the regulation of doctors, and healthcare professionals are now under much greater scrutiny than ever before. The introduction of the Government White Paper *A first class service*[1] highlighted risk management and accountability as becoming increasingly important to all members of NHS staff, from nurses and doctors through to the managers.

The purpose of this pocket-sized book is to provide a readily available practical guide and a source of comfort in times of need. It provides the background to the legal issues but the emphasis is on giving clear step-by-step guidance through a wide spectrum of legal dilemmas. It is aimed at:

- all grades of doctors in all branches of medicine, but it will probably prove particularly useful to those working in Accident and Emergency and Paediatrics, and to forensic medical examiners and general practitioners
- all grades of nurses, in all specialties
- dentists
- paramedics
- staff working in professions supplementary to medicine, for example radiographers, pharmacists, physiotherapists and chiropodists

- police officers, particularly custody sergeants
- hospital executives and managers
- lawyers in medicolegal practice.

Please note that the masculine gender has been used throughout the book except where it would be obviously inappropriate but most situations apply equally to both genders. This is not intended to cause offence in any way and is used simply to ease reading.

References

1. Department of Health. A first class service: quality in the new NHS. London: DOH, 1998

Contents

BRITISH LEGAL SYSTEMS

INTRODUCTION

There are three different legal districts in the United Kingdom – England and Wales, Scotland and Northern Ireland. Each has a separate legal system with its own hierarchy of courts and mostly, its own laws. The UK Parliament enacts laws for all areas except Scotland, which now has its own Parliament. Legislation is drafted by the Home Office, then approved by Parliament and applied by the courts. The House of Lords hears appeals for all districts except for criminal cases from Scotland. The Lord Chancellor is head of the judiciary system whereas the Home Secretary holds the responsibility for criminal policy. There is therefore a separation of powers and this independence is continued throughout the legal system. Each magistrate and judge is expected to make an independent decision, based on the facts of the individual case and they are only subject to control by other courts during the process of appeal.

CATEGORIES OF LAW

CRIMINAL LAW

Criminal law involves the public interest and it usually relates to a crime that directly and seriously threatens the well-being of the general population (e.g. crimes against the person, property or public safety). Although there is often only one victim, the prosecution is usually brought on his behalf by the Crown Prosecution Service as the outcome affects the population as a whole. Under the *Prosecution of Offenders Act 1985,* a private individual can institute a prosecution but this is rare. The object of criminal law is punitive.

CIVIL LAW

In contrast, civil law is essentially a private matter and the injured party (the claimant) usually initiates proceedings. There are four main subdivisions:

1. **Family law,** e.g. marriage, divorce and child welfare
2. **Property law,** e.g. patents, trusts and wills
3. **Contract law,** e.g. sale of goods, loans, partnerships and insurance
4. **Law of torts,** e.g. actionable wrongs such as medical negligence and defamation.

The object of civil law is compensation.

Note that some incidents may result in both criminal and civil proceedings, for example a road traffic accident may result in a criminal prosecution for dangerous driving then a subsequent civil case for personal injury.

OTHER BRANCHES OF LAW

- **Admiralty law** – this applies to both British and foreign vessels and is mostly concerned with civil matters.
- **Service law** – this applies to all serving members of the Navy, Air Force and Army and is administered through courts martial. Its role is to preserve discipline and is additional to ordinary law.
- **Industrial law** – this is concerned with conditions of employment, trade unions and industrial relations.
- **Ecclesiastical law** – this is concerned with the regulation of church affairs and control over church buildings.

SOURCES OF LAW

COMMON LAW

Common law is also known as case or judge-made law as it derives from judgements made in decided cases. It originated in the 13th century, when it began to replace the individual local systems of justice. It has been criticized for its inconsistency but it is flexible and can reflect current changes in society. It is one of the world's major systems and countries practising it include the USA, Canada and Australia. The doctrine of precedent means that lower courts are bound by earlier decisions made by higher courts and the process tends to be a step-by-step progression from one decided case to another. Since 1966, the House of Lords has declared itself free of its own earlier decisions but all decisions made by the House of Lords are binding on all but the Scottish courts. Although the Scottish courts are not bound, a decision made by the House in a civil appeal is usually regarded as highly persuasive if the case involves principles common to both legal systems. Decisions of other English and Scottish courts also do not bind each other but again they may be persuasive, particularly if they involve UK statutes.

STATUTE LAW

Statute law is that enacted by Parliament and although it may redefine and declare common law principles, statute always supersedes common law. Interpretation of statute is often very difficult although the *Interpretation Act 1978* may help and it is a key role for the judge. Where there is a conflict between two different statutes, the later one prevails. Legislation may also be made under European Communities treaties and any regulation is directly applicable without implementation or adoption by national law.

JURIES

Juries have been part of the legal system since the 12th century but they are now rarely used in civil cases and are only obligatory in serious criminal cases in Crown Courts or above. They usually consist of 12 members of the public and if they cannot come to a unanimous decision, the judge can direct them to arrive at majority decision where not more than two can disagree. In Scotland, juries are composed of 15 people selected by ballot from the electoral roll and they only ever need to reach a majority verdict. In criminal cases, the jury decides only on the verdict but in civil cases they also fix the level of compensation. Doctors can claim exemption from jury service, as can MPs and members of the armed forces. Members of the legal profession, the police, the clergy and those suffering from certain types of mental illness are ineligible. Jurors receive travelling expenses and a small subsistence allowance although they can apply for an allowance if they can prove financial loss as a result of their service.

THE LEGAL SYSTEM OF ENGLAND AND WALES

COURTS

A simplified representation of the court system of England and Wales is outlined in Figure 1.1.

MAGISTRATES

There are two types of magistrate:

- **Lay justices** – these are part-time and unpaid, with no legal qualifications. They try the majority of minor criminal offences as a 'bench'of three and are appointed by the Lord Chancellor. They must attend at least 26 sittings per year and live locally. They can only sit if they have a legally qualified clerk to assist them, to advise on the law and procedure although he must not influence their decision. The clerk is paid and is usually a barrister or solicitor.
- **District judges** – until the *Access to Justice Act 1999*, these were known as stipendiary magistrates. They are paid, legally qualified with at least 7 years of experience and can preside on their own.

JUDICIARY

The judicial hierarchy within the UK is outlined in Figure 1.2.

A judge starts as an Assistant Recorder, having been a barrister or a solicitor for a minimum of 10 years. With experience and training, they become Recorders, with an

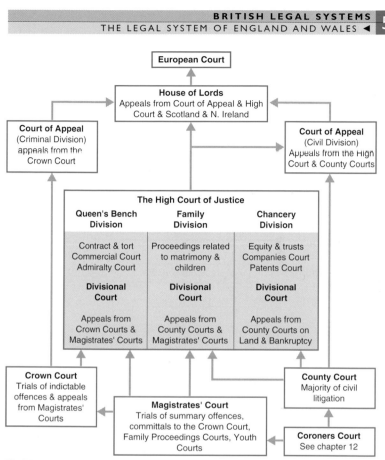

Fig 1.1 A simplified representation of the court system of England and Wales

obligation to sit in a Crown Court for at least 20 days per year. There are six circuits in England and Wales. Some then go on to become circuit judges, which is a permanent post. They can only become High Court judges by invitation. All judges are independent and self-employed. They can only be dismissed for misconduct and must be unbiased and apolitical.

CIVIL COURTS

Magistrates' Courts
These have only limited civil jurisdiction in civil cases, including adoption, guardianship and other aspects of child welfare.

County Courts
There are 226 County Courts in England and Wales, each having its

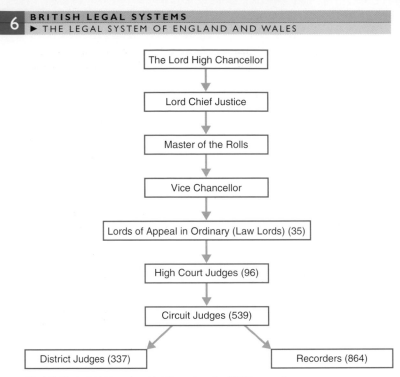

Fig 1.2 The judicial hierarchy with UK numbers for 1999 in parentheses

own geographical district. Each has at least one circuit and one district judge, dealing with cases such as building or tenancy disputes, divorce, sexual or racial discrimination, insolvency, personal injury and professional negligence. The *Small Claims Court* deals with cases valued at less than £3000 (£1000 for personal injury cases). They are heard informally before a district judge and legal aid or costs are not allowed.

High Court
This sits in London and has both criminal and civil functions. A High Court judge presides alone for most cases but he is usually joined by a jury for cases alleging libel, slander, malicious prosecution or unlawful imprisonment. The High Court is divided into:

- *Queen's Bench Division* (includes the Commercial and Admiralty Courts) – civil, commercial, admiralty and administrative law. This deals with actions relating to contract or tort; it also has a role in criminal proceedings (see below). Note that a personal injury may be a tort (negligence) or a breach of the contractual duty of care.

- *Chancery Division* (includes the Companies and Patents Courts) – company and insolvency law. The Divisional Court hears appeals from the County Courts on matters relating to disputes over land and bankruptcy.
- *Family Division* – family law, including divorce, legitimacy, wardship and adoption. The Divisional Court hears appeals on family matters from the County and Magistrates' Courts.

CRIMINAL COURTS

Magistrates' Courts

All criminal cases start here and 93% also end here. Note that the maximum sentence that can be passed by a magistrate is 6 months for one offence or 1 year for two or more either-way offences. The maximum fine is £5000. If the magistrate believes that the seriousness of the offence warrants a longer sentence, then he can commit the defendant to the Crown Court for sentencing. The Magistrates' Court also decides:

- if the defendant should be remanded in custody to await trial or be released on bail
- if the defendant should be granted legal aid
- the mode of trial as there are three categories of offence:
  — *Summary* – these are only tried in Magistrates' Courts without a jury, e.g. common assault, minor theft or motoring offences
  — *Either way* – these are offences that can be heard in either the

Magistrate's or Crown Court, e.g. theft or actual bodily harm
— *Indictable* – e.g. rape and murder. These are heard in Crown Court and the only role of the Magistrates' Court is to conduct a preliminary investigation to decide if there is a case to answer. If there is, then the defendant is committed directly for trial to the Crown Court under Section 51 of the *Crime and Disorder Act 1998* without committal proceedings.

Youth Court

This was established under the *Criminal Justice Act 1991* and replaced the term 'juvenile court'. It tries offenders aged between 10 and 17 years, unless it is an offence punishable in an adult court by a minimum of 14 years' imprisonment. These are heard in the Crown Court.

Crown Court

This was introduced under the *Courts Act 1971* and forms part of the Supreme Court of Judicature with the Court of Appeal and the High Court of Justice. Trial in the Crown Court is known as trial on indictment. A judge and jury preside and there are three tiers:

1. *Queen's Bench Division (QBD) of the High Court* – this tries Class 1 offences such as murder and treason; High Court judges preside. The Divisional Court also hears appeals on criminal cases from the Crown and Magistrates' Courts.

2. *Second tier courts* – these have either QBD or circuit judges; they try Class 2 offences such as rape and manslaughter.
3. *Third tier courts* – these have either circuit judges or recorders; they try Class 3 offences such as grievous bodily harm or fraud.

APPEALS

Criminal procedures and appeals are outlined in Figure 1.3.

- A person convicted by a Magistrates' Court can appeal to a Crown Court against:
  — sentence if the plea was 'guilty'
  — sentence or conviction if the plea was 'not guilty'.
- Appeals against Crown Court convictions are heard by the Criminal Division of the Court of Appeal:
  — from the defendant on the length of sentence and on questions of fact and law
  — from the prosecution on points of law where the accused has been acquitted.
- There is also a civil division of the Court of Appeal, which hears appeals from certain tribunals and the County and High Courts.
- The final appeal court for both civil and criminal cases is the

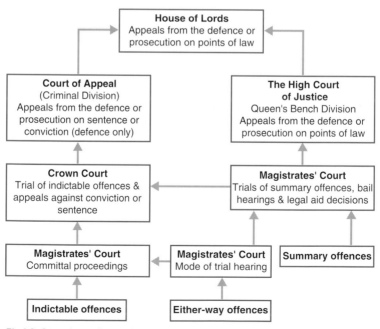

Fig 1.3 Criminal procedures and appeals

House of Lords but this only hears appeals on points of law and then only in cases where there is public interest in the outcome.

- If there is an issue concerning the interpretation of community law, then the case must be referred to the European Court of Human Rights for a ruling.

THE LEGAL SYSTEM OF SCOTLAND

English law derives from the Norman Conquest, which Scotland effectively avoided so there are significant differences between the two systems.

JUDICIARY

Criminal law is administered by a Public Prosecutor known as the Lord Advocate, who with the Solicitor General and 12 Advocates-Depute (known collectively as the Crown Counsel) prosecutes before the High Court of Justiciary on behalf of the Crown. The Crown Office is equivalent to the Lord Chancellor's department but also has a function similar to that of the Crown Prosecution Service. Both examine the evidence in serious criminal cases to decide whether or not the case should go to trial and the level of court in which it should be held.

Scotland is divided into six regions called Sheriffdoms and each has a Sheriff Principal. He is responsible for the conduct of the courts and for hearing appeals on civil matters. The public prosecutor in the Sheriff and District Courts is known as the Procurator Fiscal, who also has a parallel role to the English Coroner. He is a legally qualified member of the civil service whose

role is to assess the evidence in each case and decide whether or not to proceed with the case. The Fiscal acts as the prosecutor in summary cases but in the High Court his role is as solicitor to the Crown Counsel.

COURTS

A simplified representation of the court system of Scotland is outlined in Figure 1.4.

Stipendiary Magistrates' Court

One magistrate hears minor criminal cases and can impose a maximum fine of £5000 or 3 months imprisonment or 6 months for a second or subsequent conviction. There is currently only one court, which is based in Glasgow.

District Court

This is the Scottish equivalent to the Magistrates' Court. One or more Justices of the Peace hear minor cases and the maximum penalty is 60 days imprisonment or a fine of £2500.

Sheriff Courts

There are 49 Sheriff Courts and the presiding judge is known as a Sheriff. There are three main

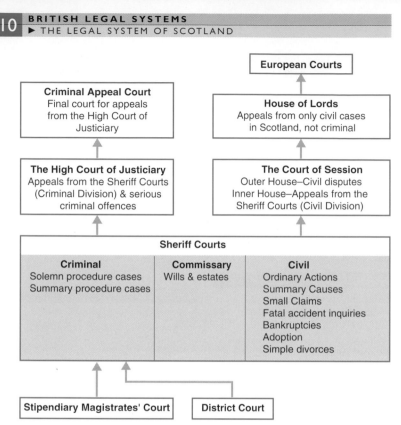

Fig 1.4 A simplified representation of the court system of Scotland

categories of work: civil, commissary and criminal.

Civil

The Sheriff Courts deal with the majority of civil litigation including adoption, uncontested divorces, company liquidations and fatal accident inquiries (see Ch. 11). There is no financial limit and there are three different types of case:

● *Ordinary Action* – e.g. divorce, property disputes, damage claims over £1500 and child welfare

● *Summary Causes* – e.g. rent arrears and debts between £750 and £1500

● *Small Claims* – e.g. minor disputes and debts under £750.

Commissary

This mainly involves the disposal of a deceased person's estate.

Criminal

Criminal cases are brought under one of the following procedures at the discretion of the Procurator Fiscal:

- *Solemn Procedure* – this is used for serious cases where the penalty involves a fine of more than £5000 or imprisonment for 3 or more months. The case is heard before a Sheriff and a jury and the Sheriff can refer the case to the High Court for sentencing as the maximum penalty that he can impose is 3 years' imprisonment.
- *Summary Procedure* – this is used for lesser cases and they are heard by the Sheriff alone. The maximum sentence that can be imposed is 3 months or a fine of £5000.

Court of Session

This is the supreme civil court and is based in Parliament House in Edinburgh. It is divided into two Houses:

- *Outer House* – this hears more serious civil disputes in the first instance, e.g. medical negligence cases. All cases are prepared and decided by judges called Lords Ordinary. They sit alone but are subject to review by at least three other judges from the nine judges who form the Inner House.
- *Inner House* – this reviews decisions made by the Outer House and hears appeals on civil cases from the Sheriff Courts.

The High Court of Justiciary

This is the supreme criminal court, also based in Edinburgh. It has the same judges as the Court of Session but they are called Lord Commissioners of Justiciary and wear different robes. The High Court cannot appeal to the House of Lords. More serious criminal cases (e.g. rape and murder) are heard before a judge and jury and, unlike the Court of Session, the High Court also sits in other towns using Circuit judges. Appeals from the Sheriff Courts are always heard in Edinburgh by a bench of three or more judges.

THE LEGAL SYSTEM OF NORTHERN IRELAND

This is very similar to that of England and Wales.

SUPERIOR COURTS

The practice and procedure of these Courts is essentially the same as their equivalents in England and Wales and they are all under the jurisdiction of the British Parliament.

Court of Appeal

This comprises the Lord Chief Justice and two Lord Justices of Appeal and sits in the Royal Courts of Justice in Belfast. It has the power to review all civil law decisions of the High Court and all criminal law decisions in the Crown Court.

High Court

This comprises the Lord Chief

Justice and five other judges and again sits in Belfast. It has a Queen's Bench Division, which deals with most civil law matters, and a Chancery Division for trusts, estates, wills and land matters. It hears more serious criminal and civil cases and appeals from the County Courts.

Crown Court

This deals with all serious criminal cases as in England and Wales. Note that terrorist offences are tried in this court without a jury and the accused have an automatic right of appeal against both conviction and sentence.

INFERIOR COURTS

County Courts

These deal with civil law and are presided over by one of 12 County Court judges. They differ from their mainland equivalents in that they also hear appeals in both criminal and civil cases from the Magistrates' Courts.

Magistrates' Courts

These are presided over by a resident magistrate who is legally qualified and similar to the stipendiary magistrates. They deal mainly with minor criminal cases and have a very limited civil jurisdiction, mainly related to family law.

Useful websites
English and Welsh courts:
www.courtservice.gov.uk
Scottish courts:
www.scotcourts.gov.uk

CHAPTER 2

LEGAL PROCEDURE AND APPEARING IN COURT

INTRODUCTION

Any healthcare professional who has had experience in the Accident & Emergency department is likely to be asked to appear in court at some point in their career. Other healthcare professionals may unfortunately become the subjects of civil litigation for alleged negligence and yet others may decide to become expert witnesses. There are many good books on the subject for those who decide to become experts (see Further reading) but this chapter aims to make the process less daunting for those for whom appearance in court is a rare occasion.

THE LEGAL PROFESSION

- *Legal executives* work for solicitors doing some of the routine work. They may have law degrees but the majority learn their trade through work experience. They may gain further qualifications through the Institute of Legal Executives (ILEX).
- *Solicitors* are legally qualified through either a law degree (LLB) or through a postgraduate qualification called the Common Professional Examination (CPE). They do a further year of study and examinations called the 'Legal Practice Course', then spend 2 years as a trainee in a firm before being made a partner. The majority of solicitors work in private practice and deal with different aspects of the law, such as conveyancing, family law, divorce, wills, estates and business law. Their role in criminal law is to protect and advance the legal rights of the accused. They advise their client and may represent him in lower courts. Solicitors can also take a test to act as an advocate in higher courts.
- *Barristers* are self-employed and can only be engaged by solicitors, not the public. After gaining the LLB or the CPE, trainee barristers must take the Bar Vocational Course for 1 year then spend a further year as a pupil of a senior barrister. Barristers give advice on points of law and procedures and represent their client in court. They are also known as Counsel and wear wigs and gowns.
- *Judges and Sheriffs* – see Chapter 1.
- *Coroners and Procurators Fiscal* – see Chapter 11.

PROCEEDINGS AT AN INQUEST OR FATAL ACCIDENT INQUIRY

See Chapter 11.

CIVIL LITIGATION

Civil cases are heard in the County and High Courts in England and Wales and in Sheriff Courts and the Court of Session in Scotland (see Ch. 1) but about 96% settle before going to court. Personal injury cases valued at more than £50 000 can start in the High Courts but most start in the County or Sheriff Courts as there is no limit to the damages that they can award. Civil cases are usually heard before a single judge but there is a right of trial before jury in cases alleging slander, libel, malicious prosecution or false imprisonment.

Actions usually begin with the injured party (claimant) consulting a solicitor, who collects information and advises his client if he believes that there is a case to answer. This may include a preliminary report by an expert. The solicitor then sends a Letter of Claim, warning the defendant of litigation if settlement is not reached. The defendant is then served with a claim form and if he fails to respond, the claimant may be entitled to a judgment by default. If the defendant does respond, then the following may occur:

1. The claimant discontinues his action.
2. The parties reach agreement (settle) before going to court. This may involve arbitration or alternative dispute resolution (see below).
3. The court decides there is no defence and judgment is made for the claimant.

4. The case goes to trial. The burden of proof is on the claimant (see below) and the standard is lower than that of criminal cases in that it is the *balance of probabilities*, i.e. which account is more likely to be the true version of events. The claimant must show:
   — that the defendant was responsible for his loss or damage (liability)
   — that if liability is established, the amount of damages that are due to compensate him for his loss (quantum) or that other measures (e.g. an injunction) are necessary. Quantum is set either by a standard book or by the jury in jury trials, often following advice from an expert witness.
5. Both parties can appeal the judgment.

ARBITRATION

This is an adjudication process that operates outside court, where a third party reviews the case and makes a decision that is binding on both parties. In the County Court, it is imposed automatically on defended cases where the claim is less than £1000. It is less formal than court proceedings, although witnesses may be called to give evidence. It offers a quicker solution but legal aid is not available. If the claim is for more than £1000, the parties can still opt for arbitration and may choose their own arbitrator.

ALTERNATIVE DISPUTE RESOLUTION (ADR)

This is another alternative to civil litigation, where a third party acts as a mediator but his decision is not binding and the disputing parties must negotiate their own settlement. If they cannot reach an agreement, then they may go on to arbitration. This process is useful if the parties wish to retain a working relationship.

CRIMINAL PROCEEDINGS

The system used for criminal proceedings in the UK is adversarial and the burden of proof is on the prosecution, i.e. they must prove that the defendant is guilty by calling evidence to support their case. The defence then tests the evidence and attempts to prove that it is not reliable and does not prove guilt to the required standard. If the defendant mounts a defence (e.g. provocation or self-defence), then the prosecution must also disprove that. The standard of proof is *beyond reasonable doubt*, i.e. the magistrates or the jury must be convinced that the defendant is guilty. Rarely, the evidential burden can shift to the defence if a specific defence is raised (e.g. a plea of insanity or diminished responsibility) but in such cases the standard is lowered to that of civil proceedings, i.e. the *balance of probabilities*.

THE PROSECUTOR

In England and Wales, the Crown Prosecution Service (CPS) brings the majority of cases. This was created in 1986 by the *Prosecution of Offences Act 1995* and conducts all police-initiated prosecutions. The CPS engages barristers to conduct the prosecution in the higher courts but CPS solicitors may act as advocates in the lower courts. The Scottish equivalent is the Crown Office (see Ch. 1) and in the High Court, the Lord Advocate or one of his Deputes conducts the prosecution. In the Sheriff and District Courts, this is done by the local Procurator Fiscal or one of his Deputes. In England and Wales, cases are brought as *R* (Regina) *v N* (name of defendant); in Scotland they are *HMA* (Her Majesty's Advocate) *v N*. Other public prosecuting authorities include the Customs & Excise, the Serious Fraud Office and the Inland Revenue. Individuals may also bring private prosecutions but this is very rare.

THE DEFENDANT

The defendant may also be known as the accused and if he pleads guilty, then no evidence is called and there is no trial before sentencing. The judge may decide to hear from the prosecution and defence in order to decide sentencing – this is known as a

'Newton hearing'. If the defendant admits his guilt to his legal representative but then pleads not guilty, he is entitled to a trial to test the evidence to prove his guilt but he cannot mount a defence.

Children younger than 10 years (child) cannot be prosecuted as they are presumed incapable of committing criminal acts but they can if they are aged between 10 and 14 years (young offender). However, the prosecution must prove that they committed the offence *and* that they were aware that what they were doing was wrong. Cases involving young offenders less than 18 years of age in England and Wales must be heard in the Youth or Crown Court but there are no special courts for young offenders in Scotland.

ARREST AND PROSECUTION

Under the *Police and Criminal Evidence Act (PACE) 1984*, a police officer may arrest anyone that he 'on reasonable grounds, suspects is about to, or is in the act of or has committed an arrestable offence'. The person must be told that he is under arrest and given the reasons for it. He must also be reminded of his right to remain silent. However, as the court may now draw an adverse inference from this silence, he must also be cautioned that it may harm his defence if he does not mention when questioned something that he may later rely on in court. The person is then taken to the police station to be charged if there is sufficient evidence, or detained for the purposes of

gathering such evidence, including interview on tape. The manner in which the detainee is treated while in the police station is strictly regulated under *PACE 1984.*

The detainee has certain rights and entitlements, including the right to free independent legal advice, to read the Codes of Practice and to have someone informed of his arrest. The detainee is then:

- released with no further action or a formal warning.
- charged and released with a caution from the police inspector.
- released on (un)conditional bail pending further investigation.
- charged and released on bail as above with a date to appear in court.
- detained for further questioning.
- charged and detained to appear before the Magistrates' Court if there are reasons that he should not be given bail, e.g. breach of previous bail conditions or no fixed address.

The action taken depends on a number of factors, including the nature and seriousness of the offence, the circumstances and the degree of intent. The investigating officer prepares the case notes and sends them to the CPS or the Fiscal, who decides whether or not to prosecute. For serious cases in Scotland, the decision rests with the Crown Counsel, based on a report from the Fiscal. In these cases, he must make his own investigations, interview witnesses and gather evidence.

The decision in all cases depends on the:

1. *Evidential test* – there must be sufficient evidence to provide a 'realistic prospect of conviction'. If not, the CPS or the Fiscal can direct the police to carry out further enquiries or discontinue the case.
2. *Public interest test* – it must be in the public interest and that of the victim to proceed with the case, for example use of a weapon or assault on a public servant, e.g. a healthcare professional or police officer.

The defence solicitor can also make representations against prosecution.

The CPS, Crown Office or Fiscal can discontinue a case at any point in the proceedings but if it is decided to proceed, then details of the charges and the evidence upon which they are based are given to the accused. The Scottish equivalent is a *complaint,* which is served by the Fiscal. The offence with which the accused is charged is important as it must reflect his conduct and obtain a conviction with adequate sentencing powers. The solicitor then prepares the defence, including interviewing witnesses and instructing experts to counteract those for the prosecution. The nature of the defence and any alibi evidence must be disclosed to the court. There are very strict rules regarding disclosure as contained in the *Criminal Procedure and Investigations Act 1996* and the *Criminal Procedure (Scotland) Act 1995* (see Ch. 6). In Scotland, more serious cases are set out in a *petition* to the Sheriff, who grants a warrant for the detention of the accused.

In cases where it is not deemed necessary to arrest the offender, e.g. following an investigation by the Inland Revenue, he will be issued with a summons. This advises him that he is believed to have committed an offence and gives him a date to appear in court.

MODE OF TRIAL

This depends on the category of offence. In England and Wales, there are three categories:

- *Summary* – these may only be heard in the Magistrates' Court, e.g. common assault, minor driving infractions.
- *Indictable* – these can only be tried before the Crown Court, e.g. rape or murder, but the accused must first appear in the Magistrates' Court for a committal hearing. This allows the magistrates to decide if there is sufficient reliable evidence to allow the jury to convict, i.e. to act as a filter.
- *Either way* – these can be heard in the Crown Court or the Magistrates' Court and the decision is made at a mode of trial hearing, where the magistrates hear representations from both the prosecution and the defence. Defendants can request a Crown Court hearing, but not Magistrates'. If the decision is made for a Crown Court hearing, then the case goes before a committal hearing as for indictable offences.

Note that the Magistrates' Court also decides if the accused should:

- be released on bail or remanded in custody to await trial
- receive legal aid – this is based on both a means test and whether it is in the public interest for him to receive it.

In Scotland, the categories of offence are:

- *Summary* – these are dealt with by the Fiscal and are heard before the Sheriff Court.
- *Solemn* – these are more serious cases and are heard initially in the Sheriff Court for a judicial examination, where the accused can answer the allegations and the prosecution can cross-examine him. The accused must then either be released on bail or remanded to custody (if accused of treason or murder, or if the Crown objects to bail). If he is held in custody, the prosecution must serve him with an indictment, outlining the allegations, list of witnesses and the evidence within 80 days or he must be released. Trials of less serious cases are also heard in the Sheriff Court before a jury but the Sheriff can refer the case to the High Court for sentencing. Very serious cases (e.g. rape or murder) are heard before the High Court.

SEATING ARRANGEMENTS

- The Judge/Sheriff/Magistrate/ Justice of the Peace sits at the head of the courtroom on a raised platform, commonly known as the Bench.

- The Clerk of Court sits in front of the Bench and is often accompanied by the stenographer.
- Counsels for the prosecution and defence sit facing the Bench, with their instructing solicitors or representative from the CPS sitting behind them. Defence counsel usually sits at the side closest to the jury but this varies.
- The jury sits to the side of the Bench, usually on the right.
- The defendant sits facing the Bench, behind the prosecutor in an area commonly known as the Dock.
- Witnesses stand on a raised platform known as the Witness Box or wait outside until the Usher calls them. In Scotland, the equivalent to the Usher is the Court Officer or Macer (High Court).
- Members of the public sit in the public gallery, which is usually at the rear of the court.

ORDER OF PROCEEDINGS

In the Magistrates' Court, the case is tried before a 'bench' of three lay justices or one stipendiary magistrate. They are responsible for reaching the verdict and sentencing where necessary. In a Crown Court, the trial takes place before a judge and jury. The jury decides the verdict but the judge has responsibility for the sentencing. The judge may only question the witness in order to clarify a point and may not cross-examine.

In Scotland, cases are heard in the High Court by a judge and jury as for the Crown Court. In the Sheriff Court, there is one Sheriff (with a jury in more serious cases); in the District Court, there is usually one Justice of the Peace but there may be more.

The prosecutor in England and Wales is the counsel for the CPS for all courts. In Scotland, High Court cases are prosecuted by an Advocate Depute and Sheriff Court cases by the Procurator Fiscal. The order is the same in the civil courts, but the counsel for the claimant replaces the prosecutor.

The chronological order of proceedings is as follows:

1. Where present, the jury is sworn in.
2. The charge is read to the defendant and he is asked whether he pleads guilty or not guilty.
3. The prosecutor makes his opening speech to outline his case (not Scotland).
4. The prosecutor calls and questions the witnesses for the prosecution. This is known as 'examination-in-chief'.
5. The defence may cross-examine each witness, either to undermine the evidence or to elicit other, more favourable evidence.
6. The prosecutor can then re-examine each witness but for the purposes of clarification only – he may not introduce new topics.
7. The defence may then make a submission of no case to answer.
8. The prosecutor has a right of reply.
9. If the submission succeeds, the defendant is acquitted.
10. The defence may (but rarely does) make his opening speech.
11. The defence calls and questions the witnesses for the defence.
12. The prosecutor may cross-examine each witness as for (4).
13. The defence may re-examine each witness as for (5).
14. The prosecutor may be allowed to call rebuttal evidence.
15. The prosecutor makes a closing speech (except in the Magistrates' Court).
16. The defence may make a closing speech if he did not make an opening one.
17. The judge or Sheriff sums up the facts and the law to the jury if present.
18. The jury or magistrates give their verdict. Note:
    — In England and Wales, the jury verdict should be unanimous, although a majority verdict of 10:2 may be accepted if the jury cannot reach agreement after a second period of deliberation. In Scotland, the jury verdict is by a simple majority of at least eight.
    — In England and Wales, the verdict can only be guilty or not guilty. In Scotland, there is a third option of 'not proven', where the accused is acquitted but has not been proved innocent.
19. The judge, Sheriff or magistrates decides sentence.

This may occur now or at a later date after the judge has received reports. Some offences carry statutory sentences, others depend on the discretion of the judge and may be influenced by factors such as past offences, mitigating circumstances and time already spent in custody.

EVIDENCE

There must be sufficient evidence to prove the case for the prosecution; this can be oral, written or in the form of objects. Only 'facts in issue' and evidence relevant to them (circumstantial) are admissible. For example for a rape case, the 'facts in issue' are:

1. Sexual intercourse must have occurred (*actus reus* = the act)
2. The accused must have known or was 'reckless' to fact that it was without consent (*mens rea* = the intention).

The circumstantial evidence could include DNA and semen samples.

Types of evidence
- *Direct* evidence is that which requires no mental processing by the judge or jury, e.g. an eye-witness account.
- *Circumstantial* evidence requires the judge or jury to draw inferences; e.g. motive, opportunity or fingerprints.

- *Hearsay* evidence is reported speech, e.g. witness statements.

WITNESSES

There are three types of witness:

- *Witness of fact* – he gives factual evidence, i.e. what he heard, saw or read. He is not paid but he may claim his travelling expenses.
- *Professional witness* – he also provides factual evidence but can give some opinions. He usually gives evidence relating to something he has seen in the course of his job, e.g. Accident & Emergency doctor. He is paid a fee related to the time that he has been in court, plus travelling expenses.
- *Expert witness* – he provides both fact and opinion evidence. His role is to guide the court over matters that are the subject of special expertise.

As a healthcare professional, you can be required to appear as any type of witness. For example, in a case where the defendant has been alleged to have committed actual bodily harm, you may be a:

- witness of fact – if you saw the act committed
- professional witness – if you treated the victim for his injuries
- expert witness – if you are an expert in the causation of different types of injury.

APPEARING IN COURT

REQUIREMENT TO ATTEND

CRIMINAL CASES

You should receive a letter from the relevant Criminal Justice Unit (CJU) or Fiscal's office, giving you the court and the time and date(s) on which the case is due to be heard. You will also be given the name of the defendant but as it is most likely that you will have seen the victim, you may have to contact the CJU or Fiscal so that you can obtain the relevant notes and read your copy of your statement (see Ch. 3). You will be asked to confirm in writing that you will be available to attend. If you do not reply or refuse to attend without good reason, then the prosecution and/or defence can apply to the court for a witness summons or citation (Scotland). This is a written order, which is served on you personally and demands your attendance. If you ignore the order, you risk being arrested and taken to court where you may be fined and/or imprisoned as a result! The CJU or Fiscal's office will usually telephone you the night before the hearing to confirm the time and the court number. You can ask them if they are prepared to take a contact telephone number and to ring you only if you are actually needed to attend. Cases are often postponed or dismissed at very short notice or it may be agreed that your statement can be read to the court, making your attendance unnecessary. However, if you do make this request, remember that it is solely for your convenience so you must be easily available and able to get to the court with the minimum of delay.

CIVIL CASES

Your instructing solicitors will usually ask you if you are willing to attend voluntarily. If you refuse or do not reply, they can obtain a witness summons as above.

PREPARATION FOR COURT

- If it is possible, familiarize yourself with the court layout, preferably by visiting it prior to your date of attendance.
- Attend a training course on giving evidence.
- Practise giving evidence in front of colleagues and ask for feedback.
- Decide in advance the strong points in your evidence, i.e. those that the judge, jury or magistrates need to know to make a reasoned decision. These are your strengths and you should return to them as often as possible, even if the question does not really relate to them. This is particularly important if you are an expert witness.
- Dress smartly. Remember that the magistrates or jury do not know you and will judge both you and

your evidence by your appearance.

- Bring your contemporaneous notes and any relevant X-rays, photographs, etc. with you as:
  — you can refer to them while giving your evidence although if you do, the opposing party has a right to see them
  — if you do not bring them, you can be sent back to retrieve them, which is both humiliating and time consuming.
- Bring a copy of your statement. You will not be allowed to refer to it in court but you should read it again before you go in.
- If you are an expert witness, bring a clean copy of your report. You will be allowed to refer to it in court but only if there are no annotations.

ARRIVAL AT COURT

- Arrive on time or slightly early as Counsel may wish to talk to you before you give your evidence
- Give the Witness Service your name and that of the trial for which you are a witness
- Ask the CPS or Fiscal's Office for a copy of your statement if you do not have one
- Ask the Usher how you should address the judge or magistrate or use Table 2.1.
- If you are appearing as a professional witness or a witness of fact, you will not be allowed to enter the courtroom before you give evidence and will be

directed to the waiting area. If you are an expert witness, you will usually be allowed to sit in the court in England and Wales but only with the leave of the court in Scotland.

GIVING EVIDENCE

CRIMINAL CASES

- On entering the witness box, you will be sworn in. You will be asked by the Court Usher (or the Judge in Scotland) if you wish to swear on the bible or other holy book or to give the oath of affirmation

> ⚠ The penalties for perjury (lying while under oath) are severe.

- You must give your evidence orally unless the opposing party agrees that your written statement can be read out, i.e. they do not wish to cross-examine you on what you have written.
- You will then be asked your name, current post, qualifications and relevant experience. It is useful to memorize the first paragraph of your statement (see Ch. 3), as it looks more impressive to give the information as a whole without being asked for it piecemeal. Remember that you are trying to convince the jury or magistrates that you are a professional person with sufficient qualifications and experience to make your evidence valid, reliable

TABLE 2.1 Correct forms of address

Court	Who sits?	What do I call them?
England & Wales		
Magistrates' Court	Magistrate	'Sir' or 'Madam'
	Justice of Peace	'Sir' or 'Madam'
Crown Court	Circuit judge	'Your Honour'
	Recorder	'Your Honour'
	High Court judge	'Your Lordship/Ladyship' or 'My Lord/Lady'
County Court	District judge	'Sir' or 'Madam'
	Circuit judge	'Your Honour'
High Court	High Court judge	'Your Lordship/Ladyship' or 'My Lord/Lady'
Court of Appeal	Lord Chief Justice	'Your Lordship/Ladyship' or 'My Lord/Lady'
House of Lords	Lords of Appeal	'Your Lordship/Ladyship' or 'My Lord/Lady'
Corner's Court	Coroner	'Sir' or 'Madam'
Scotland		
District Court	Magistrate	'Your Honour'
	Justice of Peace	'Your Honour'
Sheriff Court	Sheriff	'Your Lordship/Ladyship' or 'My Lord/Lady'
Court of Session	Lord Ordinary	'Your Lordship/Ladyship' or 'My Lord/Lady'
High Court of Justiciary	Lord Commissioners of Justiciary	'Your Lordship/Ladyship' or 'My Lord/Lady'
Fiscal Court	Procurator Fiscal	'Procurator Fiscal' or 'Sir' or 'Madam'

and significant. Do not use abbreviations: give your qualifications their full title, source and the date on which you obtained them, for example. 'I obtained the FRCS, which is the Fellowship of the Royal College of Surgeons, in London in 1993'.

- Speak slowly, clearly and loudly enough for the judge and jury to hear you easily. Use everyday language or the judge or counsel will constantly interrupt your train of thought to ask you to explain what you mean.
- Remember to ask the judge if you can refer to your notes. They

almost invariably agree but you must ask.

- Your own counsel will examine you, usually by taking you through your statement or expert report.
- You will then be cross-examined by the opposing counsel. Remember it is his job to introduce reasonable doubt so he may try to discredit both you and your evidence. It is very difficult not to take this personally but you should think of it as a compliment that he considers your evidence to be so crucial to the case!
- Do not be concerned if you have

to keep repeating your answer – barristers will frequently ask the same question, phrased in different ways, in the hope of eliciting new or different information.

- **Never** volunteer information!
- Use the questions to return to the strengths of your evidence.
- You may then be re-examined by your own counsel, but only for the purposes of clarification.
- You must address your answers to the jury or magistrates so stand facing them, turn to face counsel when he asks you a question, then turn back. This technique also makes it more difficult for counsel to interrupt you!
- The judge can only ask you questions to clarify a point and you must answer him directly.
- If counsel asks you a question that you do not understand, is unclear or too convoluted, you can appeal to the judge for clarification. Refer to the barrister as 'counsel'. The judge will then ask him to either rephrase the question or withdraw it unless he feels that it was a fair question, in which case he will direct you to answer it.
- Never speak directly to the barrister or argue with him – you will lose!

Witness of fact
Remember that as a witness of fact, you cannot give opinions.

Professional witness
As a professional witness, you may be asked for your opinion but take care not to stray out of your field of expertise: it is far better to admit that

you do not know something than to be made to appear to be a liar or stupid!

Expert witness
If you are an expert witness, then you have been called specifically to give evidence of both fact and opinion.

Your *factual* evidence has two parts and you must clearly identify the source:

- Your own observations, e.g. if you have been asked to examine the victim of an assault
- The facts that you have been told in order to prepare your report, e.g. a copy of the original Accident & Emergency notes.

Your *opinion* evidence involves the conclusions that you have reached using your specialist expertise and past experience after considering the facts.

Remember that your report is privileged, i.e. accessible only by the instructing solicitor and his client. If the solicitor feels that it might be prejudicial to his client's case, he can conceal it. However, if the solicitor does decide to use it at trial, then it must be revealed to the other side at disclosure and the privilege is lost. Note that privilege applies *only* to reports prepared for litigation purposes.

The opposing party will have had access to your report early in the case so be prepared for some rigorous cross-examination.

Remember that Rule 35 of the *Civil Procedure Rules 1998* states that your role as an expert witness is to help the court and this overrides any obligation to the party paying you.

CIVIL CASES

The process is essentially the same as that in criminal cases:

- The claimant's case is heard first.
- If the defendant is insured, his insurance company will usually run his case. For a healthcare professional, it will be run by either the Trust solicitors or his defence society; for a hospital or Trust, it will be run by the Trust solicitors (see Ch. 9).
- If you are an expert witness, you will probably be asked for your opinion on both liability and quantum to assist the judge in his final decision.

AFTER GIVING EVIDENCE

- Stay in the witness box until you are given leave by the judge.
- Check that you are released from court. You may be asked to remain in court to hear subsequent evidence, advise counsel on opposing medical opinion or be recalled to give further evidence.
- If you have appeared as a professional witness, make sure that you have been given a claim form as you are entitled to a fee and your travelling expenses, whether you have given evidence or not.
- If you are an expert witness, you should negotiate your fee with the solicitor before accepting his instructions and have it confirmed in writing. If the case is legally aided, then you must complete a claim form from the Crown Court office.

Further reading

Bond C, Solon M, Harper P. The expert witness in court – a practical guide. Crayford: Shaw, 1997

Useful websites

Courts in England and Wales: www.courtservice.gov.uk
Scottish courts: www.scotcourts.gov.uk

CHAPTER 3

PREPARING A POLICE STATEMENT

THE PURPOSE OF A STATEMENT

In the majority of cases where you have been asked to provide a statement, you will have seen the alleged victim of an assault. There is no legal obligation to complete a statement, but there is an ethical and, for some doctors (e.g. forensic medical examiners) a contractual obligation to do so. In criminal cases, statements are made under Section 9 of the *Criminal Justice Act 1967*, Section 102 of the *Magistrates Courts Act 1980* and Rule 90 of the *Magistrates Courts Rules 1981*. Your statement will be required to:

- inform the investigating officer of your findings and any treatment given
- form the basis of your factual evidence as a professional witness
- be used by the prosecuting counsel as a guide for his examination-in-chief
- be used by the defence counsel as a guide for his cross-examination
- confirm the chain of evidence in relation to forensic samples and examples (see Ch. 4).

Complete all statements at the time that they are requested. The case may be unnecessarily delayed if you do not.

WRITING A STATEMENT

GENERAL PRINCIPLES

The same rules should apply to a statement as writing clinical notes. A statement should be:

- accurate
- legible
- complete
- impartial
- understandable
- based on fact, not opinion.

For obvious reasons, a typewritten statement is vastly superior but if it must be written by hand, then it is essential that it is legible. Any errors should be corrected manually by a single line

drawn through in ink and then initialled.

⚠ Do not use correction fluid as this may lead to allegations that the statement has been altered to the detriment of either the accused or the victim!

The police supply form MG11 for statements in England and Wales or 38/36 in Northern Ireland but it is neither mandatory nor necessary to have your signature witnessed. If you have a computer, you may find it useful to design your own template but it must contain the following statement:

> This statement, consisting of x pages, each signed by me, is true to the best of my knowledge and belief, and I make it knowing that, if it is tendered in evidence, I shall be liable to prosecution if I have wilfully stated in it anything which I know to be false or do not believe to be true.

WRITING A STATEMENT ON BEHALF OF SOMEONE ELSE

If the investigating officer is unable to contact the doctor who saw the victim of an alleged assault, then he may ask you to write a statement based on the notes made at the time. This is obviously not an ideal situation and many doctors do not feel able to provide such a statement. However, this may mean that the police cannot pursue the case as they do not have written evidence of any injuries and this would be unfair to the alleged victim. There should be no adverse sequelae to making a statement based on the notes of another doctor so long as it is made clear that you never saw the patient yourself and that the quality and extent of the statement is entirely dependent on that of the original notes. It is actually documentary hearsay and can only be made admissible as evidence under the *Criminal Justice Act 1988* by the inclusion of the following paragraph:

> The medical notes were created or received by (name of examining doctor) in the course of his medical profession and the information contained in the notes was supplied by (name of examining doctor) who had or reasonably supposed to have had personal knowledge of the matters dealt with therein.

> Dr (name) is unable to make a statement as...

CONTENT

Your statement should contain specific details about yourself and the patient and also follow certain procedures, as follows.

YOUR EMPLOYMENT AND QUALIFICATIONS

Always start a statement with a paragraph about you: your name, grade or post, place of employment, your qualifications and from where

they were obtained. If you do have any specialist knowledge relevant to the case, this should also be noted. This paragraph gives your statement credibility and makes it less likely that you will be asked to appear in court.

THE PATIENT'S NAME AND AGE

Always state the name and age of

your patient so there is no possibility of mistaken identity. It may also be useful to note the sex of the patient if it is not immediately obvious from the name.

> ⚠ **Never include either your own or the patient's address! The opposing side may see your statement.**

DAY, DATE, TIME AND PLACE OF YOUR EXAMINATION

Be specific about writing the day, date, time and place of your examination so there can be no confusion. Use the 24-hour clock at all times. Also state the name and role of anyone else present, for example a chaperone or relative.

CONSENT

You should state that you obtained *informed* consent from the patient for both the examination and for preparation of the statement. **Never** write a statement unless you have seen written confirmation that the patient agrees to disclosure of the clinical notes. This should be attached to the request for the statement. Consent for examination is less important as consent can be implied from the fact that the patient came to see you for treatment (see Ch. 5).

THE REASON FOR THE EXAMINATION

Give the reason why you examined this patient. It is particularly

important to note whether or not this was solely for treatment of injuries sustained or whether there was a forensic element to the examination. Some patients will present to you purely for documentation of their injuries and may have only come because they have been advised to do so by the police.

ANY REPORTED HISTORY

Although this is hearsay evidence (see Ch. 2), it is often useful with regard to explaining the reason for the examination and your findings. Every assault is alleged until proved otherwise but a statement such as 'Mr X told me that he had been hit with a hammer but only on the head' incriminates no one while explaining why you only examined his head.

FULL DETAILS OF YOUR FINDINGS

Write everything in your statement that you wrote in your notes but use lay terms wherever possible. Remember that it is unlikely that either the investigating officer or the judge will be medically qualified and you do not want to put yourself in the position of being called to court merely to explain what you meant by an obscure medical term. Negative findings are often as important as the positive in statements as they may refute a false allegation. Remember to measure wounds and give those measurements (see Description of injuries). Unless you are an expert, you are not allowed to express an opinion in court regarding causality so do not give one in your statement. If you offer an opinion, you risk being discredited in court when opposing counsel asks you about your previous experience, qualifications and the background upon which you based your inference. The investigating officer may ask you what you think but you are not legally obliged to answer nor should you.

⚠ **Never give an opinion as to the possible cause of the injury or the likely weapon even if requested to do so!**

FORENSIC SAMPLES

List any forensic samples as shown in Chapter 4.

TREATMENT GIVEN

Investigating officers are often very interested in the type of treatment that a victim required as it can give them some indication of the severity of the injuries sustained. To a lay person, a patient that required admission would appear to be more severely injured than one that could be discharged with analgesics and this can impress a judge or jury more than lengthy descriptions of the actual injuries. The type of injury will also influence the charge and can change 'actual bodily harm' to 'grievous bodily harm'. This has far-reaching consequences for the final sentence handed down.

SIGN THE STATEMENT

This is possibly the most important part of writing a statement, as an unsigned statement is inadmissible in court. Note that this first page must be signed twice and each subsequent page must also be signed. The signature does not need to be witnessed.

COMPLETE THE REVERSE OF THE STATEMENT FORM

The reverse of form MG11 asks for contact details and dates to be avoided. Never give your home address or telephone number but it is helpful to give the hospital or your practice address and telephone number. It is also useful to give any dates when you know you will not be available (e.g. holiday) although you will be asked to provide these details again if the case goes to court. Note that this side is not included when the statement is copied for the defence lawyers.

TAKE A COPY

Make sure that you retain a copy of the statement for your own records. Cases may come to court months or even years later and although the police should provide you with a copy, it is useful to keep your own. It should be kept in a secure place and if it is a computerized record, then it should preferably be kept at your place of employment as it is then subject to the rules of the *Data Protection Act 1998* (see Ch. 6).

COMPLETE THE FEE NOTE

Complete the fee note and take a copy, as it is your only record of when you completed the statement and to whom it was sent. There is a statutory fee for each statement provided of £29.80 but there are often delays in payment and you may need to pursue the police station involved.

> ⚠ You will be expected to pay tax on all fees received so be sure to keep accurate records!

DESCRIPTION OF INJURIES

When recording injuries in your clinical notes, it is beneficial to draw a diagram in order to record precisely the site of the injury. This is particularly important when there are multiple injuries. However if you refer to any diagrams in your statement, they have to be produced as exhibits using your initials followed by consecutive numbers (e.g. 'VGM/1'). You might therefore prefer to describe the injuries in text form and this will be made easier and more accurate by applying the following rules when writing both your notes and statements.

Recording injuries

- Group descriptions according to anatomical site and note the number at each site
- Describe the position of wounds in relation to fixed anatomical points
- Describe the colour and shape of all injuries
- Accurately measure all injuries
- Use the correct descriptive term for each injury

GROUP DESCRIPTIONS ACCORDING TO ANATOMICAL SITE

Ideally, injuries should be documented in a sequential order, starting at the head and working distally to the feet. Injuries should be grouped, for example all injuries to the right arm should be described together even if they are different types of injury. Record the number of injuries so there is no confusion and no injuries are missed.

DESCRIBE THE POSITION OF WOUNDS IN RELATION TO FIXED ANATOMICAL POINTS

The position of a wound should be related to a fixed anatomical point such as the elbow, knee or umbilicus. This allows the wound to be more accurately documented, for example 'an incised wound on the forearm 10 cm from the elbow on the palmar surface'. Be particularly stringent while looking for defence wounds. These include cuts on the hands, especially between the fingers and over the palms, and an isolated transverse fracture of the ulna is a defence wound until proved otherwise.

DESCRIBE THE COLOUR AND SHAPE OF ALL INJURIES

Never try to age bruises. There have been many publications on the subject but visual ageing of bruising remains an inexact science. The most that can be said is that a bruise with any degree of yellowing is almost certainly at least 18 hours old.[1] It is essential to record any active bleeding and whether or not there are any signs of healing. A moist wound is likely to have occurred some time in the preceding 24 hours whereas a scabbed wound is probably older. Shape is best described as simply as possible (e.g. crescentic, V-shaped or irregular).

ACCURATELY MEASURE ALL INJURIES

All injuries should be accurately measured using a ruler or measuring tape. Metric units are the system of choice but imperial can be used. It is more important that the system used is consistent throughout the documentation.

USE THE CORRECT DESCRIPTIVE TERM FOR EACH INJURY

Use terms that have both legal and forensic significance (see Table 3.1 for examples). If you are forced to use a specialized medical term, you must try to explain what it means

TABLE 3.1 Terms of legal and forensic significance	
Medical term	Lay term
Erythema	Redness
Petechiae	
Abrasion	Graze or scratch
Contusion	Bruise
Haematoma	
Laceration	Burst wound
Incised wound	Stab or puncture
Slash or cut	
Periorbital haematoma	Black eye
Bite	Bite

but it is better to use lay terms wherever possible for the reasons given earlier.

Erythema or redness

Erythema is caused by pressure and can be patterned, reflecting the overlying clothing. It disappears after about 24 hours and may warrant a photograph, particularly if it outlines an apparent cause of the injury such as the imprint of a hand.

Petechiae

Petechiae are caused by arteriolar rupture and are pinpoint haemorrhages less than 2 mm in diameter. They are associated with congestion and asphyxia so are commonly found in the head and neck of victims who have suffered a strangulation attempt. Petechiae are most easily seen in the mouth and the eyes where they may be associated with retinal and subconjunctival haemorrhages. They may also be caused by suction and the characteristic 'love-bite' is actually a collection of petechiae.

Abrasion or graze or scratch

Although clinically only a minor wound, abrasions can have enormous forensic significance, particularly where the victim is dead. Abrasions are superficial skin injuries that do not penetrate the full thickness of the epidermis although they may bleed due to corrugations of the dermal papillae. They are caused by a tangential dragging or fractional force so the end opposite to the point of impact shows heaped-up epidermis (Fig. 3.1). This means that the direction of force can be deduced, for example for victims of hit-and-run accidents.

Contusion or bruise

Bruises are subcutaneous haemorrhages caused by a blunt force. Like erythema, they can be patterned and may reproduce the weapon responsible (e.g. the sole of a shoe). However, the bleeding may track under the skin, leading to confluence and loss of the pattern. It is important to note that the size of the bruise does not necessarily reflect the degree of force applied nor the size of the object used to

inflict it. Bruises tend to be larger where the skin is lax or if there is underlying bone. There may be no bruising at all in areas where the skin is thick or closely applied to the underlying tissues such as the palm or the soles of the feet. (This is the principle behind a form of torture used in Turkey called 'Falaka' where the soles of the feet are beaten with sticks. It is excruciatingly painful yet leaves barely a mark.) The amount of bruising is also affected by other factors such as age, sex, concurrent illnesses and bleeding diatheses. Patterns of bruising are often more significant, an example being fingertip bruises. These are circular or oval bruises 1–2 cm in diameter, classically found over the limbs or neck where they denote that a gripping force has been applied. It is important to distinguish bruising from other innocent causes of skin discoloration such as blue naevi, Campbell de Morgan spots and cyanosis.

Haematoma

This term is often thought to be synonymous with 'bruise' but they are not the same. A haematoma is a palpable collection of blood, usually

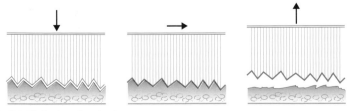

Fig. 3.1 Mechanism of an abrasion

in muscle, that may require surgical drainage.

Laceration or burst wound

This is probably the most erroneously used medical term of all. A laceration is a full thickness tear in the skin caused by a perpendicular *blunt* force – it is *not* the same as a cut or incised wound, as shown in Table 3.2.

Lacerations are most commonly found over bony prominences such as the scalp, eyebrow or elbow. They are gaping, irregular wounds, often with associated bruising or grazing. They can be linear and sometimes may be differentiated from an incised wound only by the edges. Lacerations are often dirty wounds but their most striking feature is the presence of tissue bridges. These occur because lacerations vary in depth so some elements of the subcutaneous tissue are left intact whereas others are not. The shape of

a laceration may indicate the agent responsible, for example hammers cause crescentic wounds (Fig. 3.2). They are rarely self-inflicted, as they are so painful.

TABLE 3.2 Differences between a laceration and an incised wound

	Laceration	Incised wound
Cause	Blunt force	Sharp object
Edges	Ragged and irregular	Clean and straight
Bruising?	Yes	No
Abrasions?	Yes	No
Depth	Variable	Usually uniform
Tissue bridges?	Yes	No
Position	Usually bony prominences	Anywhere
Foreign bodies?	Frequent – often dirty	Usually clean unless caused by glass

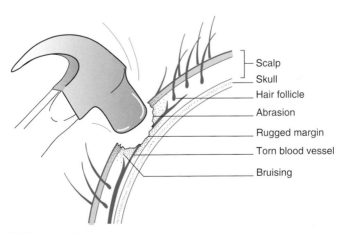

Fig. 3.2 Mechanism of a laceration

Scalp
Skull
Hair follicle
Abrasion
Rugged margin
Torn blood vessel
Bruising

Incised wound

Incised wounds can be subdivided into stab or puncture wounds and cuts or slash wounds. A stab wound is deeper than it is long whereas a slash wound is longer than it is deep. Incised wounds are usually clean, linear and of uniform depth (Fig. 3.3). They are caused by sharp objects and the shape of a stab wound can sometimes give an indication of the type of object used to inflict it, although the appearance also depends on other features such as the direction of skin tension. Slash wounds rarely reproduce the dimensions of the weapon well. Annotation of the site of an incised wound is vital as, unlike lacerations, incised wounds can be self-inflicted to support a false allegation. Multiple, superficial slash wounds in easily accessible areas on the opposite side to the dominant hand are especially suspicious, particularly in the presence of old similar scars and a psychiatric history.

Bite

Bites vary from being classical crescentic wounds with either a central pallor or petechiae (indicating sucking) and tooth marks to unremarkable bruises. It is very important to note the position, shape and size as these points can distinguish a human bite from animal, and adult from child in abuse cases.

FIREARM INJURIES

Firearm injuries can be subdivided by either the type of missile or the type of weapon.

Missile

There are two types of missile: high velocity (faster than the speed of sound) and low velocity (slower).

High velocity missiles
High velocity missiles (e.g. from a rifle) cause a permanent cavity but the high-energy transfer also causes surrounding cavitation with

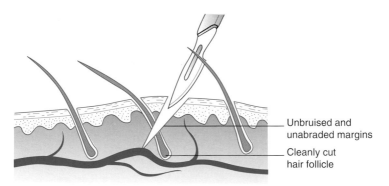

Unbruised and unabraded margins

Cleanly cut hair follicle

Fig. 3.3 Mechanism of an incised wound

ischaemia and visceral rupture. All missile wounds are contaminated but high-energy transfer wounds require aggressive debridement as they are particularly susceptible to anaerobic infection.

Low velocity missiles

Low velocity missiles,(e.g. from a handgun) cause a permanent cavity through crushing and laceration but the damage is limited to the wound track. Such injuries are only fatal if a vital organ is damaged.

Weapon

There are also essentially two types of weapon: smooth bore and rifled.

Smooth bore weapons

Theses include shotguns which fire small pellets that emerge as a solid mass then disperse. The resultant wound depends on the distance of the body from the muzzle of the gun. Contact wounds are usually circular with surrounding bruising, laceration and blackening from smoke. As the distance increases, the central wound size becomes smaller with surrounding satellite puncture wounds. Exit wounds are rare.

Rifled weapons

These include revolvers, rifles and pistols. They have parallel spiral ridges inside the barrel that cause the bullet to spin, giving it a straight flight path and characteristic scratches that are unique to each gun. The entry wounds are usually neat round holes, unless the bullet strikes at an angle, with a surrounding abrasion; contact wounds may also show charring. Exit wounds are usually much larger, with everted, lacerated margins. Note that the calibre of the bullet cannot be judged by the size of the wound.

Reference
1. Langlois NEI, Gresham GA. The ageing of bruises: a review and study of the colour changes with time. Forensic Sci Int 1991;50: 227–238

Further reading
McLay WDS. Clinical forensic medicine, 2nd edn. London; Greenwich Medical Media, 1996

Useful websites
Association of Police Surgeons: www.apsweb.org.uk
Metropolitan Police Force: www.met.police.uk

CHAPTER 4

FORENSIC SAMPLES

INTRODUCTION

Forensic samples can prove vital to the final outcome of a case but the quality of the evidence that they provide is dependent on both their collection and analysis. Anything below the highest standard can lead to miscarriages of justice, such as the case of the Birmingham Six[1] where the convictions were based on prosecution evidence that traces of nitroglycerine had been found on the accused. The tests were done using the now-defunct Griess test and the possibility of innocent contamination was not considered. The Birmingham Six were jailed in 1975 and their convictions were not quashed until 1991 so they may have suffered 16 years of wrongful imprisonment.

This chapter will focus on the collection of forensic samples, as this area can involve the healthcare professional. Under the current provisions of the *Police and Criminal Evidence Act (PACE) 1984*, the *Prisoners and Criminal Proceedings (Scotland) Act 1993* and the *Road Traffic Act 1988,* samples can be taken only by 'medically qualified personnel', i.e. doctors. However, this may change with the increasing introduction of custody nurses.

USES OF SAMPLES

DNA PROFILING

DNA profiling was introduced in 1986 using the multilocus probe technique (MLP), which was a significant advance on the conventional blood grouping techniques. MLP was highly discriminating but poorly sensitive, requiring relatively large amounts of chromosomal DNA. It was replaced by the single locus probe method (SLP), which was more sensitive and could be used on smaller amounts of material. However, SLP was less discriminating and it was often necessary to combine the results of several independent SLPs. In 1994, the Forensic Science Service (FSS) launched a new method of DNA profiling based on the polymerase chain reaction technique (PCR), whereby a targeted area of DNA can be induced to clone itself by controlled cycles of heating and cooling. This method of DNA profiling analyses areas of DNA called short tandem repeats (STR). The level of discrimination has now risen to the chance of a random match being less than one in several million and STR results can be obtained from minute amounts of chromosomal DNA (e.g. saliva on envelope seals). In the custody setting, DNA is obtained using buccal swabs and the profiles can be ready in less than 48 hours.

In 1995, the national DNA Database was established and changes to *PACE 1984* meant that buccal swabs could be taken without consent by police officers from any detainee charged with a recordable offence. All samples that are suitable for DNA profiling from both suspects and crime scenes are submitted to the FSS for analysis and inclusion in the database. Suspect DNA is cross-referenced against all known crime scenes and vice versa in a continuous process. This not only links suspects to different crimes but may also reveal serial cases as it can link crimes committed by the same person, even if that person is not yet on the database. As yet, results from the database may not be used as direct evidence and the police are required to take a further sample from the suspect to be submitted in court.

A suspect may also be required to give a blood sample for the purposes of DNA profiling. This is used for:

- identification of any blood found at the scene of the crime
- exclusion of his own blood from any found on his body or clothing. This is particularly important where there has been a cross-allegation of assault.

Victims of crime may also be asked to provide a blood sample for DNA profiling but this cannot be demanded. It is used for:

- identification of the scene of the crime
- exclusion of any DNA found at the scene of the crime

- purposes of correlation with any blood found on the suspect's clothing
- purposes of correlation with any blood found on potential weapon(s).

DNA profiling has also been used in paternity suits, issues of probate, cases of alleged incest and in the identification of human remains. Analysis of mitochondrial DNA is now possible, allowing DNA profiling an even wider range of material, including hair shafts.

BIOCHEMICAL ANALYSIS

- Hair and other objects (e.g. fibres retrieved from the victim, suspect or crime scene) can be analysed for chemicals such as dyes and cleaning products.
- Swab analysis can show body fluids (e.g. semen or saliva) that can be matched to the assailant, as well as other substances (e.g. lubricants or gunpowder residue).
- Blood samples are used for DNA profiling and the detection of drugs and/or alcohol. This is particularly important for suspects detained under the *Road Traffic Act 1988* (see Ch. 16) and in cases such as so-called 'date rape', where the victim is given a sedative such as flunitrazepam (Rohypnol) prior to being assaulted.
- Urine analysis can demonstrate the presence of alcohol, drugs and/or their metabolites much later than blood analysis, for example the metabolites of cannabis are detectable in the

urine up to 46 days after ingestion.

COMPARISON MICROSCOPY

- Objects such as hair and fibres retrieved from the victim or the crime scene can be compared under the microscope with those from the suspect to see if they match.
- Nail clippings can be matched to broken pieces of nail found at the scene by matching the nail striations.

PROBLEMS WITH TAKING SAMPLES

INFORMED CONSENT

Section 62 of *PACE 1984* allows the collection of intimate samples such as blood, semen and swabs from a person in police custody but only *with his consent.* A detainee is not obliged to provide specimens for forensic examination or to undergo medical treatment or examination, except for intimate body searches (see below) but Subsection 10 of *PACE 1984* allows the court to make adverse inferences from a refusal to consent. The taking of intimate samples requires authorization from a superintendent or above. Police officers can take samples of urine and saliva and perform external swabs, including mouth swabs. Any others are classed as intimate samples and must be taken by a registered medical practitioner. The detainee must be 17 or more in order to give a valid consent. If he is 14–17, then consent must be obtained from both the detainee and a parent or legal guardian. If he is younger than 14, then consent should be obtained from the parent or legal guardian only.

It may be very difficult to be certain that you have obtained informed consent, i.e. that the person fully understood the reasons for providing the samples and the possible future ramifications. This is particularly true for samples for blood alcohol and drug analysis as, by definition, the person is considered to be under the influence of drugs and/or alcohol. If in doubt, ensure that you have a witness to the fact that you have given the person a full explanation and make a full and detailed record of the conversation. If you doubt the capacity of the person to give consent through reason of mental illness or impairment (see Ch. 5), then either ask for a psychiatric assessment or take the samples in the presence of an 'appropriate adult' to help explain and oversee the procedure. **Never** take samples from an unconscious patient as this cannot be justified as being in the 'best interests' of the patient (see Ch. 5) except in *very exceptional circumstances* such as the comatose victim of a serious assault and even this is subject to debate. **Never** take samples by force if you cannot obtain consent.

CONTAMINATION

Locard's principle is as follows:

> Every contact leaves a trace

This means that trace evidence can be accidentally transferred from one object or person to another so you should never examine or take samples from both the parties involved in one incident. This is particularly true for cases that rely heavily on the forensic evidence for a conviction. In a murder case, the doctor who pronounced life extinct in the victim must never then examine the possible suspect. In a rape case, the suspect should never be examined at the same location as the victim by the same doctor or transported in the same vehicle.

CONTINUITY OF EVIDENCE

TAKING SAMPLES

The samples required depend on the type and nature of the crime committed. You should discuss this with the investigating officer prior to taking any samples but if in doubt, take the sample as there is unlikely to be another opportunity. Before taking any samples, check that the requesting officer has read out the correct part of the request for intimate samples as stated in *PACE 1984* and note that the Act states that intimate samples may be taken only by a medically qualified practitioner. For blood samples obtained under the *Road Traffic Act 1988*, there is also a section that must be read out by the sergeant to both you and the detainee prior to the sample being taken.

Make sure you write that you have taken informed consent and take all the samples in the presence of the requesting officer. If you are taking blood, always swab the venepuncture site with an alcohol-free swab and use the forensic kits where available. You should label all your samples and place them in a tamper-evident bag, which is then labelled with the same details. Sign the bag then hand it to the requesting officer who will seal and also sign it.

It is important to note that some of the provisions of *PACE 1984* do not apply in Scotland. Under the *Prisoners and Criminal Proceedings (Scotland) Act 1993*, a "police constable can, with the authority of an inspector or above, take hair by cutting or combing, as well as fingernail scrapings and any external swab of the body using reasonable force if necessary.

LABELLING

All samples and bags must be labelled in the order in which they were taken with the following:

● The name (and the date of birth) of the person providing the sample
● The hospital or custody number
● Your initials, then the number of sample (e.g. VGM/1) – this is the exhibit number
● Your name
● The place, date and time the sample was taken using the 24-hour clock.

Note that if more than person is examined from the same enquiry, then item numbers should continue in series, as there should never be two samples with the same number even if they were taken from different people on different days.

In Scotland, exhibits are known as productions.

YOUR STATEMENT

Your statement should contain a numbered list of all the samples with the:

● exhibit number
● nature of the sample
● site of the sample
● time of the sample, using the 24-hour clock
● seal number of bag

For example: 'I took the following samples:

1. VGM/1 – Wet swab taken from Mr X's right hand at 18.05 hours. Seal No.B2543218
2. VGM/2 – Blood EDTA sample taken from Mr X's left arm at 18.00 hours. Seal No. B2543219'

Always give the name and rank of the police officer to whom you handed the samples and the time at which you did so, for example 'I handed the samples to DS Smith at 18.40 hours'.

TYPES OF SAMPLES

Table 4.1 and the following text outline types of samples and their processing.

● Blood taken for the purposes of the *Road Traffic Act 1988* must be drawn as a single sample of 8 ml, then divided equally into two 4 ml samples, preferably in the standard containers provided in the FSS packs. In hospital, the single sample should be divided into two vials containing an

anticoagulant such as fluoride and oxalate (see Ch. 16).
● Blood taken for grouping or DNA analysis should be placed in a container containing a preservative such as EDTA (ethylene diamine tetra-acetic acid).
● Both urine and saliva can be collected by police officers. Urine should be collected in the vials provided by the FSS as these contain preservatives at the level

TABLE 4.1 Types of samples and their processing

Sample type	Reason for analysis	Method of sampling	Storage
Blood preserved (sodium fluoride and potassium oxalate)	Alcohol drugs and volatile substances	8 ml venous blood	Refrigerate
Blood EDTA	DNA – victim and accused	5 ml venous blood	Refrigerate
Urine preserved	Alcohol and drugs	20 ml urine	Refrigerate
Saliva	Semen if oral penetration < 2 days ago	5–10 ml saliva	Freeze
Mouth swab	As for saliva DNA	2 sequential samples by rubbing swab around mouth	Freeze
Mouth washings	As for saliva	Rinse mouth with 10 ml sterile water and retain washings	Freeze
Skin swabs	Body fluids and other substances, e.g. lubricants	Dry swab for moist stains, wet swab for dry	Freeze
Head hair	Body fluids, e.g. semen Foreign particles or fibres Control sample (suspect)	Cut or swab area Remove visible items and use either comb or tape Cut 10–20 hairs close to scalp	Freeze
Pubic hair	Body fluids, e.g. semen Foreign hairs or fibres	Cut or swab area Comb hair and collect debris	Freeze
Vulval swab	Body fluids if vaginal penetration < 7 days or anal < 3 days Lubricant if used or from condom < 30 hours	Rub 2 sequental swabs over vulval area (moisten if required). Number in order taken	Freeze
Vaginal swab – low	As for vulval swab	2 sequential swabs under direct vision before speculum is passed. Number in order taken	Freeze
Vaginal swab – high	As for vulval swab	2 sequential swabs using unlubricated speculum. Number in order taken	Freeze
Endocervical swab	Only necessary if vaginal > 48 hours previously	1 swab via the speculum	Freeze
Penile swab	Body fluids if intercourse < 2 days Lubricant if used or from condom < 30 hours	2 sequential swabs from coronal sulcus and 2 from shaft and glans. Number in order taken	Freeze

TABLE 4.1 Types of samples and their processing (con't)

Sample type	Reason for analysis	Method of sampling	Storage
Perianal swab	As for penile swab except intercourse can have occurred up to 3 days previously	2 sequential moistened swabs from perianal area. Number in order taken	Freeze
Rectal swab	As for perianal swab	Swab lower rectum after passing proctoscope 2–3 cm into anal canal	Freeze
Anal canal swab	As for perianal swab	Swab with proctoscope withdrawn	Freeze
Fingernails	Recovery of trace evidence	Cut or take scrapings with swab	Freeze

suitable for alcohol analysis. Saliva and mouth washings can go into plain, sterile tubes.

- Only plain, sterile swabs should be used and they must not be placed in transport medium.
- Wet stains are sampled using a dry swab but the swab should be moistened in distilled or tap water for dry stains. If tap water is used, then a control swab of the tap water should be provided. A further swab should be rubbed over the skin adjacent to the stain as a control sample for the skin.
- Note that many of the samples should be stored in a freezer so all containers must be shatter-proof.

- If instruments are required to collect samples (e.g. scissors or specula), then they must be sealed and disposable.
- Specula or proctoscopes can be moistened with sterile water but lubricants must never be used.
- Hair that appears to be contaminated (e.g. with semen) should be cut where possible or swabbed if the person objects. A control sample of hair should also be cut or swabbed.
- Pubic hair can be combed but never plucked.
- Nail clippings are preferable to scrapings but the nails may be too short.

INTIMATE SEARCHES

Although not strictly related to the taking of forensic samples, a request to perform a non-consensual intimate search on a detainee can cause the healthcare professional concern so it is worthy of inclusion in this chapter.

Under Section 55 of *PACE 1984*, a medical practitioner or a registered nurse can perform a non-consensual intimate body search under certain circumstances. The Act distinguishes between two groups of material for which such a search can be authorized. Section 55(a) deals with intent by a detainee to conceal dangerous weapons for use on either himself or on others while in custody, while Section 55(b) deals with drugs. Intimate searches for drugs are limited to Class A drugs in Schedule 2 of the *Misuse of Drugs Act (MDA) 1971*; these are usually heroin and cocaine. The superintendent authorizing the search must believe that the suspect has concealed drugs in a body orifice *and* that he intended to supply the drugs, which is an offence under section 5(3) of the *MDA 1971*. This is known as 'appropriate criminal intent' in *PACE 1984*. An intimate body search consists of the physical examination of the orifices including the ears, nostrils, mouth, rectum and vagina; most doctors and nurses are unwilling to perform it without consent. The medical defence organizations, the British Medical Association and the General Medical Council recommend that this be done under only very exceptional circumstances. However, there are two factors to consider before refusing:

- Section 55 also allows the search to be performed by a police officer of the same sex and the detainee may prefer that it be done by a doctor or nurse.
- The risk posed to third parties by concealed weapons or drugs.

Note that the healthcare professional also has an obligation to warn the patient of the possible complications following the ingestion of certain drugs, such as bowel obstruction and drug leakage leading to acute intoxication and possible death from overdose. The search for drugs can only be performed in suitable medical premises so it should never be done in a police station; however the search for a concealed weapon may be done at either.

Reference
1. *R v Kilkenny* [1991] 93 Cr. App. R. 287; [1992] 2 All ER 417

CONSENT

INTRODUCTION

Every person has the right to have his body integrity protected against invasion by others and only rarely can this be compromised (e.g. during arrest). Consent is the ethical precept that allows a patient to make invasion lawful – whether that invasion is into their body or their confidential information. There is no statute in UK law that applies to the general principles of consent but case law (see Ch. 1) has established that touching a patient without valid consent may constitute a civil or criminal offence.

> Every human being of adult years and sound mind has a right to determine what shall be done with his own body; *and* a surgeon who performs an operation without his patient's consent commits an assault, for which he is liable in damages.
> Justice Cardozo (*Schloendorff v Society of New York Hospital 1914*[1])

DEFINITIONS OF CONSENT

Consent can be:

- *implied* – this is behavioural, e.g. a patient voluntarily undresses for examination
- *express* – the patient gives permission orally or in writing. The form most commonly used is that published in 1990 by NHS Management Executive but it has no space for risks and complications.

All types of consent are equally valid although written consent does give documentary evidence. However, it is the *reality* of consent that is important – a consent form signed in the absence of information is valueless. Some procedures have a statutory requirement to obtain written consent and must not proceed without it, for example fertility treatment under the *Human Fertilisation and Embryology Act 1990.*

OBTAINING CONSENT

Consent is only valid if the following principles apply:

- The patient is legally competent.
- The consent is given freely.
- It is *informed,* i.e. the patient has had the intention, nature and purpose of what is intended fully explained although the extent of the information given will depend on the:
  — age and maturity of the patient
  — physical state

— mental state
— intellectual capacity
— nature of the condition
— reason for the procedure, e.g. it may be possible to give a fuller explanation for routine surgery than in an emergency
— questions asked by the patient e.g. side effects.

● It is *appropriate,* for example consent to sterilization does not include bilateral salpingectomy. Note that is only acceptable to perform additional procedures if it would not be safe to delay them, e.g. a life-saving manoeuvre. They should never be done purely for convenience.

It has always been traditional to leave the process of obtaining consent to the most junior member of the medical team but the responsibility actually lies with the clinician providing the treatment. The clinician can delegate the task to another healthcare professional but he must ensure his delegate is adequately informed, qualified and trained for the task. It should also be a continuous process that starts well in advance of the proposed procedure so that the patient has ample opportunity to review his

decision before the procedure starts.

The following information may be relevant when obtaining consent:

● Details of the likely diagnosis and any further investigations necessary or desirable
● The likely prognosis, with or without treatment
● The options available for treatment, management or palliation with details of their possible benefits, risks and probabilities of success
● The purpose and details of any proposed procedures, including side effects (see below)
● Follow-up
● The likely recovery time
● A reminder that the patient has the option to change his mind at any time and that he has the right to a second opinion.

Note

Always ask the patient if he has understood the information that he has been given and if he would like any more before he makes a decision. Answer all questions as fully and honestly as possible – if you do not know the answer, say so!

DISCLOSURE OF RISK

Patients must be given sufficient information, in a way that they can understand, in order for them to make an informed decision about their treatment. The case of *Sidaway v Board of Governors of the Bethlem*

Royal Hospital 1985[2] affirmed that the decision about what degree of disclosure of risk is best calculated to assist a particular patient to make a rational decision is a clinical judgement. However, the judge added the proviso that the decision might be subject to challenge by the courts if there is conflict between medical opinions over non-disclosure. There have now been several cases in which patients have successfully sued for negligence on the basis of failure to inform of recognized risks. Risks must now be disclosed if:

- they are *material,* i.e. a reasonable ('prudent') patient or doctor would attach significance to them
- the incidence is high, e.g. 10% risk of stroke. There is a nebulous cut-off point that suggests that a doctor does not need to inform a patient of a risk if it is < 1%
- the incidence is low but it has potentially serious consequences
- the patient specifically asks, i.e. he attaches significance to a particular risk.

However, the doctor is not under any pressure to disclose if he thinks that it would be detrimental to the patient or if the patient is unable to give consent (e.g. unconscious). This is called 'therapeutic privilege' but it should not be invoked simply because the clinician feels that the patient might be upset by the information or might refuse consent. Note that negligence claims based on flawed consent are virtually never successful in the United Kingdom.

> **Note**
>
> *Always* make a contemporaneous entry in the notes to state that consent has been obtained and write down what you told the patient – particularly a list of all the risks and complications.

If the patient wishes to give consent without hearing all the information, he is entitled to do so but this *must* be recorded in the notes and he should be given opportunities in the future to change his mind if appropriate.

LIMITS OF CONSENT

Criminal or unethical conduct cannot be made lawful just because a patient requests it. This includes:

- euthanasia
- maiming (some centres will not perform sex conversions due to this)
- non-therapeutic sterilization
- some cosmetic surgery
- experimental or unorthodox procedures.

CONSENT AND THE UNCONSCIOUS PATIENT

Medical staff can treat an unconscious patient in the absence of consent under the 'doctrine of necessity'. This means that as long as the clinician can justify his actions as being in the 'best interests' of the patient, then he will be protected against any subsequent legal action. However, the treatment can only be justified if:

● it saves life
● and/or prevents further deterioration
● and/or improves health
● it is in accordance with established medical practice
● the patient was competent and did not refuse treatment prior to losing consciousness.

The treatment must be limited to that required to satisfy the above criteria if the patient is likely to regain capacity upon recovery. Note that nobody can give consent on behalf of a competent patient so it is both pointless and technically illegal to ask a relative to sign a consent form.

> **Note**
>
> *No one* can give consent on behalf of a competent patient.

In law, there are two standards adopted for making decisions on behalf of incompetent patients: 'best interests' (objective) and 'substitutive judgement' (subjective).

'Best interests' (objective)
The decision maker must choose the treatment that would be most beneficial to the patient. This standard is mainly used for those who have never been competent but it is sometimes applied in emergency situations

'Substitutive judgement' (subjective)
The decision maker must provide the treatment that the *patient* would have chosen if he was still competent. This standard is mainly used for those who were once competent but are no longer, for example *Airedale NHS Trust v Bland 1992/3*[3] where treatment was discontinued on the basis of his feeling that it would be what he would have preferred (see Ch. 13). Substituted judgements tend to be based on quality, rather than quantity of life

CONSENT IN THE MENTALLY IMPAIRED

In England, Wales and Northern Ireland, no one can legally give consent if a patient over 18 lacks capacity through mental impairment. Treatment can be given only in the best interests of the patient in accordance with standards acceptable to a responsible body of medical opinion and preferably

involving the guardian or relatives. In some cases, it may be wise to seek guidance from the courts (e.g. sterilization in severe mental handicaps). In Scotland, people over 16 can appoint a 'tutor-dative' under the *Adults with Incapacity (Scotland) Act 2000,* who then has the authority to make medical decisions on behalf of the patient. Note that this proxy can act in all circumstances where the patient has been assessed as incompetent but he cannot demand treatment that is judged to be against the patient's best interests. There are currently plans for legislative reform in England and Wales to provide adults without capacity with a similar 'decision-maker'. However, it seems likely that treatments that are not curative, such as sterilization, abortion or organ donation, will still be subject to court approval on an individual basis.

Consent and the mentally ill is covered in Chapter 15.

CONSENT AND MINORS

In England and Wales, the *Family Law Reform Act 1969* allowed minors of sound mind and over 16 years of age to give consent to surgical, medical or dental procedures. In Northern Ireland, the relevant Act was the *Age of Majority Act 1969;* in Scotland, it is the *Age of Legal Capacity (Scotland) Act 1991*. However, in 1985, the case of *Gillick v West Norfolk & Wisbech AHA 1984–5*[4] led to the ruling that unless a statute or otherwise provides, a minor can give consent if they have sufficient understanding and intelligence to make the decision. This overrides the parental rights but the judge recommended that the healthcare professional should always try to obtain parental authority.

The ruling was confirmed in the *Children Act 1989* and the *Children (Scotland) Act 1995*, which gave statutory power to mature minors under the age of 16 to consent to treatment, although the case of *Re R*[5] in 1992 modified the concept of the 'competent minor'. R was a disturbed girl of 15 who required sedation but refused medication during her lucid phases. The local authority applied for wardship to be able to administer treatment without consent and R appealed against it. The Court of Appeal ruled that the powers of the court were wider than parental since the court could override both consent and refusal of treatment and were not affected by the *Children Act 1989*. It also said that Gillick did not apply since maturity could not be assessed where the mental state fluctuated. Therefore the order was upheld on the basis that R was not 'Gillick competent' and treatment could be authorized in her best interests. This meant that *refusal* to consent did not carry same weight as *agreement*. So far, the courts have judged that minors who refuse treatment agreed by their parents and advocated by healthcare professionals are not Gillick competent.

In England, Wales and Northern Ireland, a court or a person with parental responsibility may authorize an investigation or treatment in the child's best interests if an apparently otherwise competent child refuses. In Scotland however, only the court can do this.

As the numbers of competent children that have withheld consent to life-saving treatment have risen since the introduction of the *Children Act 1989*, there is now increasing recognition that such children do have a right to legal representation and that their views deserve proper consideration.

If the child is under 18 (16 in Scotland) and not competent, then a *competent* person with parental responsibility (see Ch. 14) can authorize investigations or treatment that are in the best interests of the child. Note that the authority of only one person is necessary for a therapeutic intervention, even if another refuses. If the intervention is non-therapeutic (e.g. male circumcision on religious grounds) and two parties disagree, then it is advisable to seek a court ruling. If that person refuses to give consent, then a clinician can still treat the child without consent if it is an emergency (Fig. 5.1). If the treatment or investigation is non-urgent but still in the best interests of the child,

then the clinician can ask either the local or the health authority to apply for a 'specific issue order' under the *Children Act 1989* (see Ch. 14). This allows the clinician to give the treatment without there being any other effects on the child's welfare as may occur with a wardship order. This is the most acceptable route to follow where the care of the child is otherwise good and the only point of disagreement is the withholding of consent, for example a child who requires blood but whose parents are Jehovah's witnesses. It is probably more appropriate for the local authority to make the application as they have a statutory responsibility to investigate and act in cases where the child may be at risk of appreciable harm, which would include the withholding of necessary treatment. Serious non-therapeutic interventions such as sterilization should always be referred to the High Court. Note that once a minor is made a ward of court, then no major treatment can be given without permission of the court.

CONSENT IN SPECIAL CASES

JEHOVAH'S WITNESSES

An adult is entitled to refuse a transfusion but a special consent form is required. The clinician must be satisfied that the patient is aware of the risks involved in his refusal and that he is not under any pressure from his relatives to make his decision, i.e. there is no coercion. If the patient has made his wishes

clear but then loses consciousness, it cannot be assumed that he would have changed his mind so a transfusion should still be withheld. The clinician must decide whether or not he is prepared to treat the patient under these circumstances, i.e. is he prepared to allow the patient to die? If not, then he can transfer the patient to the care of another clinician.

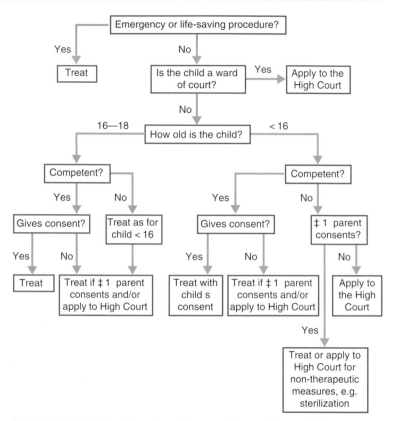

Fig. 5.1 Consent in children (where 'parent' is anyone with parental responsibility)

Minors present a much greater problem. Under the *Children and Young Persons Act 1933*, it is a criminal offence to ill-treat, neglect or abandon a child under the age of 16, so if a child dies, the result could be a charge of manslaughter. In the past, the solution used to be to make the child a ward of court, but now treatment is either instigated by the clinician, preferably a consultant, as being in the best interests of the child or given under a Specific Issue Order.

PRISONERS

Prisoners cannot choose their doctor, but otherwise they have the same rights as anyone else and consent must be obtained before any treatment is given.

INTIMATE SAMPLES

See Chapter 4.

SCREENING

Patients giving consent to screening tests should be aware of the following:

- The purpose of the test
- The likelihood of positive and negative findings
- The risks of false negative and false positive results
- Any risks associated with the screening process
- Any medical, social or financial implications, e.g. HIV tests and life insurance
- Follow-up.

CLINICAL TRIALS

The Royal College of Physicians produced guidelines on research on healthy volunteers in 1986 and guidelines for research on patients in 1990:

- Consent must be obtained on a special form that is tailored to the particular requirements of research and preferably by independent person.
- The research must be subject to an independent ethical review.
- The patient must be aware that participation is voluntary and that he can decline or withdraw without any prejudice to his future care.
- Patients without the capacity to consent should only be entered

into trials where there is likely to be a therapeutic benefit and where similar research would not be feasible on competent patients.

Legal opinion is divided as to whether someone with parental responsibility can give consent for a minor to be involved in research, particularly where the research while not in the best interests of the child, is *not against* them.

CONSENT TO POST MORTEM AND REMOVAL OF HUMAN TISSUE

See Chapter 11.

CONSENT AND DEAD PATIENTS

The executors of the will can give consent on behalf of dead person (e.g. the release of records to an insurance company) but it must be *all* the executors. If the person died intestate, then the descendants can apply for a 'letter of administration', but they must be the personal representatives of the deceased, which is not necessarily the next-of-kin.

SURGICAL IMPLANTS

Any device or prosthesis implanted surgically becomes the property of the person in whom it is implanted unless a special consent form is signed that gives rights of ownership to the Trust. After death, it forms part of the estate.

ASSESSMENT OF CAPACITY

Capacity relates not to the final decision, but to the way in which the patient arrives at that decision. A patient is deemed to be competent if he can be shown to:

1. comprehend and retain information that has been presented to him in a way that he can understand
2. believe that information
3. be able to weigh up that information and use it to make an informed decision.

Note that capacity may fluctuate and that a patient may have the capacity to consent to simple procedures, but not to more complicated ones. Remember that refusal to consent requires a higher level of capacity than agreement and that patients who suffer from mental illness do not necessarily lack capacity.

> **Note**
> If in doubt, ask for a second opinion!

It is often appropriate to ask a psychiatrist to see the patient, particularly if he is refusing potentially life-saving treatment. There is also a book called *Assessment of Mental Capacity: Guidance for Doctors and Lawyers* (see Further reading), which is very useful. Assessment of capacity may be compromised by stress, pain, alcohol, drugs or coexisting illness (e.g. head injury) and but note that in law, alcohol intoxication alone does not make a person incapable of making decisions (see Ch. 16).

REFUSAL TO CONSENT

As shown, competent patients have a right to decide whether or not to accept treatment, even when refusal might result in harm or even death. This includes the instructions contained in valid advance directives (see Ch. 13) if the healthcare professional believes that the clinical situation falls within the scope of the directive. The reasons for refusal can be rational, apparently irrational or even non-existent as long as the patient can be shown to have capacity. This is particularly difficult to accept with patients who deliberately harm themselves but if the psychiatrist genuinely believes that:

- the patient intends to commit suicide
- he was competent when making that decision
- he shows no signs of mental illness

then the wishes of the patient must be respected. However, he should be continually encouraged to accept help and asked to sign a written assurance that:

- his refusal is an informed decision
- he understands the proposed interventions
- he understands the risks and likely prognosis of refusing treatment.

If he is unwilling to sign such a declaration, then this must also be carefully noted. There are those that believe that if the patient attends a hospital, then he cannot genuinely wish to avoid treatment, but it does not necessarily follow that he is mentally ill or incompetent.

> **Note**
>
> If a patient refuses treatment and you are satisfied that he is competent and understands the consequences of his refusal, then you *cannot* assume that he would have changed his mind if he loses consciousness. You have *no right* to treat him under those circumstances and you could be successfully sued if he survives!

There are very few exceptions to the right to refuse:

Pregnancy

In 1992, there were two cases that gave the right of a viable foetus to life precedence over the right of the mother to refuse treatment. In *Re S*[6], a woman refused to have a Caesarean section on religious grounds, despite the fact that it represented the only chance of survival for her child. The court gave permission to proceed in the interests of the foetus. In *Re T*,[7] a pregnant woman involved in a car accident refused a transfusion after

talking to her mother who was a Jehovah's witness. A court order was obtained to legalize transfusion and this was upheld by the Court of Appeal. The judge said that a mentally competent adult has an absolute right to consent to treatment, to refuse it or choose an alternative unless the choice might lead to the death of a potentially viable foetus. However, in 1998, the judge in the case of *St George's Healthcare NHS Trust v S*[8] ruled that pregnant women retain the right to refuse treatment, even where it is intended to benefit the unborn child. This means that the situation is now much less clear-cut than it was.

The competent minor

A minor who has been deemed competent to accept treatment may not be competent to refuse it. The case of *Re W*,[9] in 1992 confirmed that a higher level of comprehension is needed to refuse treatment than to consent to it.

Undue influence

If a healthcare professional believes that the patient is refusing treatment because of coercion by a relative, such as in the case of *Re T* above, and the treatment is life-saving, then the consultant in charge of the patient should ask for guidance from the courts.

A competent patient is also entitled to withdraw his consent at any time, even during a procedure and this wish must be respected. However, before stopping, the healthcare professional should ascertain the problem, check that the patient's capacity has not changed and explain the consequences of abandoning the procedure. If stopping the procedure might endanger the life of the patient, then the healthcare professional is entitled to continue until it is no longer the case.

If the patient is judged to be incompetent, then he can be treated under the doctrine of necessity. If this involves detention against his will under common law, then it becomes more controversial and may lead to future litigation under the *Human Rights Act 1998*, which came into force in October 2000. This provides that no one of 'sound mind' may be detained except in some special circumstances and it remains to be seen if incapacity can be argued to equate to being of 'unsound mind'. Note also that if the patient leaves the hospital, there is no legal basis to forcing him to return (e.g. by the Police) unless he has been sectioned under the *Mental Health Act 1983* (see Ch. 15).

SITUATIONS WHERE CONSENT IS NOT REQUIRED

In the following situations, the examination can continue even if the patient refuses to give consent:

- Examination of immigrants by port and airport medical staff on entry into the United Kingdom
- Examination and/or treatment of a patient suffering from a notifiable disease (requires an order from a magistrate)
- Psychiatric examination and/or treatment under Sections 2, 3, 35 and 36 of the *Mental Health Act 1983* (see Ch. 15)
- Routine external medical examination of new prisoners to exclude infectious diseases
- Examination of dairymen and food handlers if there is a suspected outbreak of staphylococcus or salmonella
- Routine external medical examination of members of the armed forces.

Cases
1. *Schloendorff v Society of New York Hospital* 105 NE 92 (NY, 1914)
2. *Sidaway v Board of Governors of the Bethlem Royal Hospital* [1985] AC 871
3. *Airedale NHS Trust v Bland* [1993] AC 789
4. *Gillick v West Norfolk & Wisbech AHA* [1986] AC 112
5. *Re R (A minor) (Wardship: consent to treatment)* [1992] Fam 11
6. *Re S (Adult: Refusal of medical treatment)* [1992] 4 All ER 671
7. *Re T (Adult: Refusal of treatment)* [1993] Fam 95
8. *St George's Healthcare NHS Trust v S* [1998] 3 All ER 673
9. *Re W (A minor) (Medical treatment)* [1992] 4 All ER 627

Further reading
BMA. Consent tool kit. London: BMA Publications, 2001

BMA/Law Society. Assessment of mental capacity: guidance for doctors and lawyers. London: BMA Publications, 1997

Department of Health. Reference guide to consent for examination or treatment. London; DoH, 2001

General Medical Council. Seeking patients' consent: the ethical considerations. London: GMC, 1998

Useful websites
British Medical Association: www.bma.org.uk
Department of Health: www.doh.gov.uk/consent
General Medical Council: www.gmc-uk.org

CHAPTER 6

CONFIDENTIALITY AND DISCLOSURE

INTRODUCTION

Until the year 2000, there was no statutory duty of confidentiality in the United Kingdom – it was only an implied form of contract between the healthcare professional and the patient. Unauthorized disclosure of professional secrets therefore merely constituted a breach of contract and was subject only to civil proceedings. However, the *Human Rights Act 1998* came into operation in October 2000 and Article 8 states 'Everyone has the right to respect for his private and family life, his home and his correspondence', thus making confidentiality a statutory obligation.

This change in the law should not matter in practice, as confidentiality has always been an important part of the doctor–patient relationship and forms part of the Hippocratic oath:

> Whatever things seen or heard in the course of medical practice ought not to be spoken of, I will not, save for weighty reasons, divulge.

Confidentiality is an agreement that gives the confider the right to expect discretion and the confidant the right to hear the truth, but also the obligation to ensure guardianship of the information received. However, the traditional concept of confidentiality is becoming threatened by new developments, such as the Internet, which can make it more difficult for both patients and healthcare professionals to control information linkage and leakage. The Caldicott report, produced by the Department of Health in 1997,[1] identified and examined 86 different data-flows of patient-identifiable information. It made 16 recommendations about the use of data within the health service, including:

- appointment of a Caldicott guardian within each Trust to oversee issues of confidentiality (usually the Medical Director)
- establishment of a programme to reinforce staff awareness of confidentiality and information security in the NHS
- introduction of a new NHS number to replace other identifiers
- introduction of standards and protocols against which to judge the justifications for information use.

PRINCIPLES

These are set out for doctors in *Confidentiality: Protecting and Providing Information*[2] from the General Medical Council (GMC) and in Clause 9 of the United Kingdom Central Council (UKCC) *Code of Professional Conduct*[3] for registered nurses. Registered paramedics are expected to adhere to the *Code of Ethics and Professional Conduct* produced by the Ambulance Service Association. The principles are:

- All patient-identifiable health data, including medical illustrations, videos, tape recordings, photographs, X-rays, computer files, genetic registers, disease management registers, manual records or even that held only in the memory of healthcare professionals, are subject to the rules of confidentiality. Non-clinical information such as a hospital attendance or their address, is also confidential.
- Clinicians and those working in professions with access to medical data such as receptionists, paramedics and social workers have a duty to refrain from disclosing information learnt directly or indirectly in their professional capacity.
- Care must be taken when either discussing or talking to patients in public areas such as at the reception desk or on the telephone to avoid being overheard by third parties.
- Those responsible for confidential information must ensure that the information is adequately protected from improper disclosure during storage, transfer and disposal. This includes

information stored, sent or received by fax on computer and e-mail
- Record-holders are:
  — individual Trusts for NHS patients; they should confer with the consultant concerned before release
  — general practitioners
  — private clinics for private patients.
- The minimum retention period is 8 years for personal health records and 25 years for maternity and obstetric records. However the Department of Health recommends that any medical record, or summary of it, should be retained for as long as it remains relevant to the long-term care of the patient.
- Any disclosure of information must be limited to only that which is necessary and this is dictated by individual circumstance.
- The duty of confidentiality is *not* affected by the death of the patient and information cannot be released without the informed consent of *all* the personal representatives (e.g. executors of the will). Post mortem reports merit the same degree of confidentiality as a clinical examination.

EXCEPTIONS

THE PATIENT GIVES CONSENT

A clinician can disclose information if the patient gives consent to do so

but he must ensure that the patient is aware of the consequences, i.e. what will be disclosed and to whom, the reasons for any such disclosure and the likely sequelae. Consent to disclose must be given freely and is usually express but it can be implied, for example a patient under the care of more than one person such as a general practitioner (GP) and a district nurse (see Ch. 5). If the patient specifically *refuses* consent, then the clinician may not disclose the information unless it can be justified by any of the following circumstances.

DISCLOSURE IN THE PATIENT'S INTERESTS

Sharing information with other staff

Healthcare professionals can share information with colleagues to assist in the management of a patient, for example a paramedic can divulge confidential information about a patient when transferring his care to the Accident & Emergency staff. However, this information must be limited to that which might affect any future treatment. Deciding what is clinically necessary may be very difficult, particularly where the information is particularly sensitive. For example, a hospital specialist may not be able to justify telling a patient's GP that he has AIDS if the patient refuses to give consent as the condition would not place the GP at risk under normal circumstances. However, failure to disclose may put the patient at a therapeutic disadvantage and the GMC has advised that a specialist should tell the patient this while encouraging him that his GP should be informed.

If a competent patient refuses to allow his information to be shared with other healthcare professionals, it should be respected even if it may compromise his safety.

> **Note**
>
> It is the responsibility of the healthcare professional divulging the information to ensure that other professionals realize that it is confidential.

Information should not be circulated to others simply because they are healthcare professionals, and managers and administrators should not have routine access to identifiable data. Note also that a clinician who is the subject of a complaint is prohibited from seeing the notes made by a colleague involved in the subsequent care of the patient concerned unless the patient gives consent for him to do so.

Sharing information with the next-of-kin

If the patient specifically requests that the next-of-kin are not told, then his wishes must be respected *except* in exceptional circumstances, for example a patient with tuberculosis where there is a serious risk of the immediate family becoming infected. Very occasionally, disclosure to a third party may be justified if it is felt that telling the patient would be injurious to his health, such as informing him that his illness is terminal.

Disclosure in the patient's medical interests

Information necessary to allow emergency treatment of a patient may be disclosed without consent unless the patient has previously forbidden this while acknowledging the risks to himself. If a patient is incapable of giving informed consent (e.g. through immaturity, illness or mental incapacity), then information may be disclosed in the non-emergency situation to an appropriate person or authority if it is in the patient's best interests. However, the patient is still entitled to know that this is being done (e.g. a young child suspected of having suffered a non-accidental injury). Disclosure would be justified both in the child's interest and in the public interest in the prevention of child abuse. NHS staff also have a statutory duty under the *Children Act 1989* to cooperate with a social services investigation and this includes disclosure of any relevant information (see Ch. 14).

DISCLOSURE IN THE PUBLIC INTEREST

Disclosure may occasionally be justified in the public interest but, if so, it must be limited to the proper authorities or to those who may be at potentially fatal risk without the information. For example, neither AIDS nor HIV-positive status is notifiable and confidentiality must be maintained unless someone else is at risk. The GMC and the Nursing and Midwifery Council (NMC) advise that if a doctor or nurse is aware that a fellow healthcare worker is HIV positive, then he has an ethical duty to inform a senior colleague if the person refuses to inform them himself.

When considering disclosure in the public interest, the healthcare professional should:

- balance the benefits of disclosure against the potential harm
- assess the urgency of the situation
- exclude all other means of achieving the objective
- consider whether or not the subject might be persuaded to give consent unless this might make the situation worse
- inform the subject *unless* this might increase the risk of harm
- limit the disclosure to only that which is strictly necessary
- seek assurances that the information will only be used for the purpose for which it was intended
- be able to justify the decision.

Healthcare professionals who breach patients' confidentiality without consent must be prepared to justify their actions to their disciplinary bodies. However, in America, a healthcare professional may be held as being negligent if he does *not* break confidentiality when made aware that his patient poses a serious danger to another person. In a case heard in 1976,[4] the judge ruled that a therapist had an obligation to use reasonable care to protect the intended victim – to warn them or others close to them, notify the police or take whatever other steps were necessary. In 1997, changes to the 1991 *Ontario Medicine Act* made it mandatory for doctors to inform the authorities when a patient threatens serious harm to others and the doctor believes that violence is likely. In the United

Kingdom, disclosure in the public interest remains an ethical rather than a legal duty and courts are wary of claims to justify a breach of confidentiality.[5] Healthcare professionals ought to be assured of the support of their professional bodies and there is also some protection in law. The *Public Interest Disclosure Act 1998* provides protection for individuals who make certain disclosures of information in the public interest and allows them to bring action in respect of victimization.

If the police demand access to a patient's notes or enquire about attendance at the Accident & Emergency department, then the person in charge must not release the information unless they have consent from the patient or a court order. However, it should be noted that it is a criminal offence under Section 51 of the *Police Act 1964* to give misleading information as this amounts to obstruction. A senior doctor may make an exception in

cases where a serious crime has been committed; the application for release of information is made in writing by a senior police officer and where the advice in the box on this page from a case heard in England in 1990[6] can be applied.

If a patient assaults a healthcare professional, then he can inform the police even if it means telling them that the patient has been seeking medical treatment. However, the information must not contain any clinical details.

DISCLOSURE TO THE DRIVER AND VEHICLE LICENSING AUTHORITY (DVLA)

See Chapter 16.

DISCLOSURE UNDER THE DATA PROTECTION ACT 1998

The *Data Protection Act 1998* came into force on 1 March 2000, giving effect in law to the 1995 EC Data Protection Directive. It controls 'processing' of data, which includes collection, use, disclosure, destruction and storage, and forms part of the *Consumer Protection Act 1987*. It replaced and extended the 1984 Act and, applies to both computerized personal data and that held in structured manual files, which includes health records. A health record is defined as information relating to the patient made by or on behalf of a healthcare professional, including doctors, dentists, nurses, pharmacists, paramedics, chiropodists,

---

Reasons for release of information

- The risk is real, immediate and serious
- The risk will be substantially reduced by disclosure
- Disclosure is the only means by which the risk can be minimized
- The disclosure is limited to that reasonably necessary to minimize risk
- The consequent damage to the public interest in confidentiality is outweighed by the interest in minimizing risk

physiotherapists and other practitioners. This means that it has replaced the *Access to Health Records Act 1990* (see below), which formerly gave individuals the right of access to manual records that were not covered by the *Data Protection Act 1984*. There are eight principles of the Act, which are as follows.

Personal data should be:

1. Obtained fairly and lawfully and only processed if one or more of the conditions listed in Schedule 2 are met. These include the data subject giving consent, legal requirements and in the best interests of the data subject. In the case of sensitive personal data, one or more of the conditions listed in Schedule 3 of the Act must also be met. These include explicit consent and legal obligations but the Act also gives further strict controls on the actual processing.
2. Obtained for only one or more specified lawful purposes and not used or disclosed in any matter incompatible with these.
3. Adequate, relevant and not excessive.
4. Accurate and where necessary, kept up to date.
5. Not kept for longer than is necessary.
6. Processed in accordance with the rights of the data subject, which are as follows:
   — To access that data within 40 days of request (for medical records), subject to an access fee of up to £10. The patient, their personal or legal representative or anyone with parental responsibility for a minor can apply and they are entitled to an explanation of all medical terms. If the application is made by a third party, then it must be ensured that the patient is incapable of giving consent. 'Therapeutic privilege' allows the record holder to deny access if he feels that it might cause harm to the physical or mental health of the patient or if it would identify another individual, other than another healthcare professional
   — to know the source of the data and any recipients of disclosed data
   — to have inaccurate data rectified or erased where appropriate
   — to seek compensation in the event of illegal processing
   — to withhold permission to use their data in certain circumstances, e.g. mailing lists.
7. Safeguarded from unauthorized or unlawful processing or accidental loss or damage.
8. Transferred only to countries that offer adequate data protection.

Personal data means information that relates to a living individual (the data subject) who can be identified from those data. Sensitive data include race, religion, criminal history and sexual orientation.

The Information Commissioner has now replaced the Data Protection Registrar and registration has been replaced by notification. The Commissioner maintains a public register of data controllers and a general description of the type of processing performed by each data controller. Notifications are renewable annually.

DISCLOSURE UNDER THE ACCESS TO HEALTH RECORDS ACT, 1990

Under the *Access to Health Records Act 1990*, which came into force in England, Scotland and Wales on 1 November 1991, patients were entitled to have access to any non-computerized health records made after that date. The Northern Ireland Act was identical but only came into operation on 30 April 1994 and therefore only applied to records made on or after that date. The Acts have now been repealed except for the sections dealing with access to records relating to the deceased. Access can be denied if the record holder believes that the patient gave the information on the basis that it would not be disclosed to the applicant and patients can request that a note be put in the records to that effect. If the information requested relates to a claim, then the applicant may be shown the relevant parts only.

DISCLOSURE TO EMPLOYERS AND INSURANCE COMPANIES

Where assessments are performed on behalf of a third party, such as a pre-employment medical, the doctor or nurse has an obligation to release the results to the requesting employer and this may necessitate the disclosure of personal information. The potential employee must be informed of this and the potential consequences when his consent is sought for the examination. It is generally advisable to keep evidence of the patient's consent on their file. If the patient refuses to give consent, then the assessment should not be done and the refusal documented. The *Access to Medical Reports Act 1988* came into force on 1 November 1989 and applies to England, Wales and Scotland. There are separate regulations for Northern Ireland called the *Access to Personal Files and Medical Reports (NI) Order 1991*. These Acts give a patient the right of access to any medical report prepared for insurance or employment purposes by a practitioner who *is or has been responsible for his care* and therefore *applies only to reports prepared by the patient's own general practitioner*, not occupational physicians or nurses. The Acts also allow the patient to withhold consent, request amendments or stop the report. The patient can be refused access if the GP believes that the report might endanger his physical or mental health or that disclosure would reveal information about another identifiable person other than a healthcare professional.

CONFIDENTIALITY WITHIN THE FAMILY

Minors

Minors may wish to conceal their medical history from their parents and if they are 'Gillick-competent' (see Ch. 5), then they do have a right to confidentiality (e.g. contraception or treatment for a sexually transmitted disease). However, the healthcare professional has an obligation to try to persuade the minor to inform his parents.

Spouses

Spouses have no automatic right to information and this includes termination of pregnancy and sterilization. Also, the healthcare professional cannot contact the police in cases of marital violence without the consent of the patient, however frustrating that may be.

DISCLOSURE FOR TEACHING, AUDIT AND RESEARCH PURPOSES

Clinical audit should ideally be carried out by healthcare professionals with clear professional obligations to maintain confidentiality but, increasingly, Trusts and GP surgeries are commissioning third parties to carry out audits on their behalf. Commissioners of such services must ensure that their employees have firm contractual obligations with regard to the preservation of confidentiality. The BMA guidelines state that the disclosure of 'truly anonymous data' for teaching, audit, research or commercial purposes does not breach confidentiality. This guidance has been challenged by the Association of Community Health Councils of England and Wales, the statutory body that represents patients interests, who feel that patients can often still be identified.

This was also the view taken by Justice Latham in a case in 1999,[7] which would have meant that individual informed patient consent would have been required for all research studies using anonymized data. This would have had potentially disastrous consequences for all future research had it not been overturned on appeal. In the past, discussion about the use of anonymized information has focused on what can be considered to be truly anonymous, for example information such as date of birth, diagnosis or postcode may not identify an individual in isolation, but can in combination. Use of minimal data identifying the patient's electoral ward, sex and year of birth is usually acceptable for administrative or research purposes but if the patient cannot be adequately anonymized, then consent should be sought. If it cannot be obtained, the information cannot be used for teaching or audit but if it is for research purposes, the ethics committee must make a decision as to whether the potential public benefit of the research outweighs the rights of the individual. The GMC advises that consent must be obtained before disclosure of any named data and that patients must be informed before their data are transferred to cancer registries in order to comply with the *Data Protection Act 1998*.

ADVERSE DRUG REACTIONS

Doctors have both ethical and legal responsibilities to report adverse drug reactions to the Medicines Control Agency (MCA) but the 'Yellow Card' system has now changed (see Ch. 7). In order to comply with the *Data Protection Act 1998* and the GMC guidelines on confidentiality, they must now give the patient's initials, age and a local identification number or code (e.g. a hospital number instead of the name, sex and date of birth). This information can still be used to cross-reference all reports and prevent duplication but there is no longer any need to get the consent of the patient.

COMPLAINTS

When investigating a complaint, reasonable efforts must always be made to obtain consent before identifiable health information is used, unless a delay would pose a risk to others. If the patient refuses to give consent then his views should be respected unless the public interest in protecting other people outweighs them. The GMC and the NMC have powers to require the production of medical records for their investigation of complaints as part of the performance procedures involving doctors and nurses (see Ch. 10).

GENETIC INFORMATION

Genetic information is bound by the same principles of confidentiality as any other but there is an added dimension in that the information may have direct relevance to other family members. This can result in a conflict for the healthcare professional between a duty of confidentiality to the patient and a duty to protect others from avoidable harm and suffering. The healthcare professional should advise the patient about the implications of the test results and encourage him to share the information with his relatives. If he refuses to do so, the healthcare professional should consider:

- the severity of the disorder
- the level of predictability of the information provided by testing
- what if any, action the relatives could take to protect themselves or to make informed reproductive decisions if they were told of the risk
- the level of harm or benefit of giving and withholding the information.[8]

If the healthcare professional still feels that he must inform the relatives, then this should be discussed with the patient and the reasons given. Wherever possible, the patient should not be identified to the relatives and if they do not wish to be told the information, it should not be forced upon them.

DISCLOSURE TO TAX INSPECTORS

Healthcare professionals in private practice may disclose confidential information to the tax inspector but every effort must be made to separate financial information from clinical records.

DISCLOSURE TO A SOLICITOR

Information regarding a patient can be released to his own solicitor but only with the patient's written consent and the notes must not relate to any other person.

DISCLOSURE OF DOCUMENTS FOR CIVIL LITIGATION

Records are usually made available for litigation purposes through the *Data Protection Act 1998* but in medical negligence and personal injury cases, application for disclosure can be made under Sections 33 and 34 of the *Supreme Court Act 1981*. These allow disclosure to the applicant and his legal or medical advisers prior to 'discovery' (the point at which all parties must produce all documents in their possession relevant to an issue in the litigation) although disclosure may be limited to the latter two only. The patient's consent is necessary and 'relevant documents' include case notes, X-rays, laboratory reports and letters but not reports prepared specially for the litigation. The record holders do not need to obtain the consent of the patient or any healthcare professionals involved, but they should be informed. This allows them the opportunity to apply to the court to

have it set aside if they so desire and circumstances permit. Section 35 of the Act gives the court the power to refuse to order disclosure if it would be injurious to the public interest. The courts may also order that an action be stayed where a patient making a claim of negligence refuses to allow access to relevant medical records.

Disclosure of audit records may present a particular problem and has led to calls for special protection.[9] There is no case law as yet but if a Trust were to bring a defence of accident or coincidence in explaining an adverse clinical incident, any audit records relating to that procedure would become disclosable. The audit process involves comparing current practice to agreed standards, so it often reveals deficiencies. The patients and the staff involved should be anonymized but it is often possible to identify people. This could both assist the plaintiff's lawyer and make staff less inclined to become involved in audit.

DISCLOSURE OF DOCUMENTS FOR CRIMINAL PROCEEDINGS AND INQUESTS

A healthcare professional in the witness box has absolute privilege and is protected against any action for breach of confidence. However, he cannot refuse to answer questions on grounds of breach of confidentiality. In criminal proceedings, if a doctor refuses to disclose health records, the person seeking the information may apply to the court for a witness summons to be issued requiring the doctor to produce the information. This is covered by the rules on third party disclosure, introduced in the *Criminal Procedure (Scotland) Act 1995* and the *Criminal Procedure and Investigations Act 1996*. The applicant must state specifically what information he requires, why it is material to the case and why he believes it is held by the third party. He must also give reasons why the doctor will not release the information voluntarily. The doctor (not the patient) then has 7 days to notify the court that he wishes to make representations, either in writing or at a hearing. If a hearing is requested, the doctor (or his representative) can bring up the issue of confidentiality or argue that the information requested is not material to the case. If, despite this, the witness summons is issued, the doctor must then provide the records or be found in contempt of court

Police investigating a serious arrestable offence (basically any offence where the penalty is 5 or more years imprisonment) can obtain a search warrant from a Magistrate under the *Police and Criminal Evidence Act (PACE) 1984* but Section 11 of the Act specifically excludes medical records and samples from the search. If the police wish access to these, then they must apply for a special order under Section 9 of *PACE 1984* and this can only be issued by a circuit judge. Such orders are given only

rarely and under very limited circumstances (e.g. stolen medical records). The doctor or health authority must be informed that the application has been made and they are given the opportunity to be heard by the circuit judge before the order is issued. The only exception to this rule is in cases where the police are investigating acts of terrorism and an order may be given without such notice under the *Prevention of Terrorism (Temporary Provisions) Act 2000*. Where possible, it is more appropriate that the records are presented as oral evidence by the clinicians who made them since the issues involved are often very complex and judges are rarely medically qualified.

Some Coroners or Procurators Fiscal have both medical and legal qualifications but if a Coroner wishes to see the medical notes he must also apply for a High Court order although healthcare professionals will usually take them to the inquest on request. Similarly, most Coroners will allow the consultant in charge of the patient to see the post mortem report before the inquest although this practice has been criticized. It has been suggested that the consultant might change the way in which he presents his evidence once given the benefit of hindsight. However, it should be borne in mind that the consultant is entitled to attend the post mortem anyway – either as a hospital representative or where information has been sworn that he is responsible for the death.

STATUTORY DUTIES

There are some statutes that require the healthcare professional to breach confidentiality under very strictly controlled circumstances:

- *NHS (Venereal Diseases) Regulations 1974* require every Trust to ensure confidentiality over records and only allow release of information in order to treat or to prevent the spread of disease. These regulations require explicit consent from patients to allow a genitourinary medicine clinic to communicate with their GP – it cannot be taken to be implied.
- The *Human Fertilisation and Embryology Act 1990 as amended by the Human Fertilisation and Embryology (Disclosure of Information) Act 1992* also requires explicit consent for disclosure of information from a fertility clinic to the patient's GP.
- Notifications under the provisions of the *Factories Act 1895* and of the *Control of Substances Hazardous to Health (COSHH) Regulations.* Employers are required to assess and control health risks arising from exposure to hazardous substances, including biological agents and body fluids, and to inform employees about them. Correspondingly, healthcare professionals must declare their immune status so their employer can protect any vulnerable workers by removing them from exposure to a quantified risk. Currently, all healthcare professionals who undertake

duties that may expose them to the risk of contracting hepatitis B must provide evidence of immunity before starting work.
- Abortions must be notified to the Chief Medical Officer under the *Abortion Act 1991.*
- Known or suspected drug addicts must be notified to the Home Office under the provisions of the *Misuse of Drugs Act 1971* and the *Misuse of Drugs (Notification and Supply to Addicts) Regulations 1985.*
- Births and deaths must be notified under the *NHS (Notification of Births and Deaths) Regulations 1982.* Note that birth and death certificates are public documents and copies can be obtained for a fee.
- Note that doctors are not under any statutory duty to report a death to the Coroner but they must complete the death certificate in such a way that any need for referral is made clear to the Registrar of Births and Deaths who is under such a duty. If they do not, they can be accused of obstructing the Coroner. If a doctor gives a false cause of death, then he can be charged under the *Perjury Act 1911* and the *Births and Deaths Registration Act 1953.* It is also illegal to omit conditions that may have contributed to the death such as HIV infection, even if it may cause distress to the relatives.
- Certain infectious diseases must be notified to the local authority

Notifiable diseases (1981)

- Acute encephalitis
- Acute meningitis
- Cholera
- Diphtheria
- Dysentery
- Food poisoning (suspected and confirmed)
- Infective jaundice
- Lassa fever
- Leprosy
- Leptospirosis
- Malaria
- Marburg disease
- Measles
- Ophthalmia neonatorum
- Paratyphoid fever
- Plague
- Rabies
- Relapsing fever
- Scarlet fever
- Smallpox
- Tetanus
- Tuberculosis
- Typhoid fever
- Typhus fever
- Viral haemorrhagic fever
- Whooping cough
- Yellow fever

(see above) under the *Public Health (Infectious Diseases) Regulations 1988* and the *Public Health (Control of Disease) Act 1984*. Note that AIDS and HIV are *not* notifiable *(AIDS (Control) Act 1987)*.

- Any person with information that might prevent an act of terrorism must inform the police (and/or the armed forces in Northern Ireland) under the *Prevention of Terrorism (Temporary Provisions) Act 2000*.

- There is a statutory duty under Section 172 of the *Road Traffic Act 1988* to give information that may identify a driver who is suspected of having committed a road traffic offence but staff should only release the name and address, not any medical information.

REMEDIES FOR BREACH OF CONFIDENTIALITY

Patients' expectations of confidentiality may be raised by the Patient's Charter which states that 'every citizen has the right of access to their health records and that those working for the NHS are under a legal duty to keep their contents confidential'. A patient can claim for damages for improper disclosure of information even if he did not suffer financially and this can be the basis of a complaint to the Health Service Commissioner (see Ch. 8). Breach of confidentiality is not defamation or slander as the information disclosed is usually true – the fault lies in the inappropriate disclosure. For a breach of confidentiality to be said to have occurred:

CONFIDENTIALITY AND DISCLOSURE

- The information divulged must be confidential
- It must have been divulged in confidence
- There must be unauthorized use of information to the detriment of the person to whom it relates.

Possible consequences for the healthcare professional include:

- *Disciplinary proceedings* – up to and including being struck off
- *Civil proceedings* – which may result in the healthcare professional having to pay the patient compensation
- *Criminal proceedings* – the introduction of a statutory duty of confidentiality in the *Human Rights Act 1998* may well give rise to such proceedings in the future

SPECIALIZED DOCTORS

Prison Doctors
Prisoners cannot choose their doctor but otherwise they have same rights as a free person and consent to treatment must be given freely.

Armed Forces Medical Officers (MO)
No MO can be required to treat a patient in accordance with a given policy when it is not in the patient's best interests. However, service personnel must accept some loss of confidentiality, for example the MO might be required to discuss cases with his Commanding Officer (CO) in the interests of the unit as a whole although these circumstances should be rare. The CO is obliged to respect the confidential nature and source of the information and the disclosure should be limited to the essential minimum. The individual should also be informed of the disclosure and the reasons why the MO considers it necessary. Informed consent to disclose voluntarily should be obtained wherever possible and the MO would be

advised to discuss the matter with his medical defence organization.

Ship's surgeons
This scenario is similar to that of an Armed Forces MO (above) as the captain must be aware of any incapacities in his crew in order to run a safe ship.

Expedition doctors
Similar to ship's surgeons.

Occupational health physicians and nurses
These are employees of the company but they still have a duty of confidentiality. If they are required to perform medical examinations, then the nature of the examinations and the need for disclosure of any findings should be set out in the contract. They should only treat or refer patients with the cooperation of the GP unless in an emergency.

Forensic Medical Examiners (FME)
It is often difficult to ensure confidentiality when examining

detainees in custody as the FME may need to be chaperoned by a police officer. It is important that the FME makes his role clear to the detainee and to obtain consent. This is particularly important when conducting an examination under Section 4 of the *Road Traffic Act 1988* where 'no part of the examination may be regarded, as confidential' (see Ch. 16). Detainees are not obliged to submit to examination or treatment nor to provide specimens, and the FME must always obtain consent or risk being sued for assault.

CONCLUSIONS

The following eight principles probably best sum up the ideal approach to the use of confidential information.

Principles of using confidential information

- Make sure you can justify the purpose
- Seek consent to disclose where possible
- Only use it when it is absolutely necessary
- Use the minimum data necessary
- Anonymize data whenever possible
- Ensure access is strictly on a need-to-know basis
- Ensure that everyone understands their responsibilities
- Understand and comply with the law

References

1. Department of Health. The Caldicott Committee. Report of the review of patient-identifiable information. London: DoH, 1997
2. General Medical Council. Confidentiality, protecting and providing information. London: GMC, 2000
3. United Kingdom Central Council. Code of professional conduct. London: UKCC, 1992
4. *Tarasoff v Regents of the University of California* 529 P 2d 55 (Cal, 1974); 551 P 2d 334 (Cal, 1976)
5. *X v Y* [1988] All ER 648
6. *W v Egdell* [1990] Ch 359, [1990] 1 All ER 835
7. Fletcher AP. Editorial – Source Informatics Ltd versus Department of Health: Appeal Court reverses judgment of Mr Justice Latham and allows use of anonymised patient information without consent. Adverse Drug React Toxicol Rev 2000; 19(1): 5–8
8. British Medical Association. Human genetics: choice and responsibility. Oxford: Oxford University Press, 1998
9. Womack C, Roger S, Lavin M. Personal paper: Disclosure of clinical audit records in law: risks and possible defences. BMJ 1997; 315: 1369–1370

Further reading

General Medical Council. Good medical practice. London: GMC, 1998

United Kingdom Central Council. Guidelines for Professional Practice. London: UKCC, 1996

Useful websites

www.dataprotection.gov.uk
www.homeoffice.gov.uk
General Medical Council: www.gmc-uk.org
Nursing and Midwifery Council: www.nmc.org.uk

CHAPTER 7

CLINICAL GOVERNANCE AND RISK MANAGEMENT

WHAT IS CLINICAL GOVERNANCE?

When the NHS was established in 1948, there was no explicit consideration given to the quality of the healthcare provided and it became apparent that the standard of care offered by the NHS varied greatly between hospitals, between departments in the same hospital and between general practices. In 1997, in the White Paper *The New NHS: Modern, Dependable,*[1] the government made it a statutory duty for all healthcare professionals to become involved in a quality agenda. This Paper set out a 10-year strategy for the NHS, with a huge emphasis on quality, and introduced the concept of corporate governance. It also promised to modernize the NHS, to improve communication and to make services quicker, more convenient and more consistent. In 1999, the National Institute for Clinical Excellence (NICE) was established, followed by the Commission for Health Improvement (CHI) a year later.

small, with a staff of about 20–30 people, and use teams of experts to produce guidance for the NHS and patients on medicines, medical equipment and clinical procedures. NICE also appraises those treatments and issues guidance on whether or not the treatment can be recommended. The impetus for NICE was to stop 'postcode prescribing' where the decision whether or not patients received treatment depended upon the policies of whichever health authority they came under. Its detractors describe NICE as an instrument for rationing healthcare as it does not have the resources to test the interventions and it has no influence on drug licensing. This means that deliberations are often based on a cost–benefit analysis and the cheapest intervention is not always the best.[2] There is also some debate that clinical effectiveness does not necessarily equate to patient effectiveness.

NICE

NICE is part of the NHS and has the status of a special health authority. It is accountable to the Secretary of State for Health and to the National Assembly for Wales. Its role is to promote clinical and cost effectiveness across England and Wales through research and the development of evidence-based guidelines. Its Scottish equivalent is SIGN (Scottish Inter-Collegiate Guidelines). Both are relatively

CHI

The role of the CHI is to promote, guide and monitor local clinical governance and the National Service Frameworks (NSF), which delineate the care that different groups of patients should expect (not applicable to Scotland). It is intended that CHI will visit every NHS trust and health authority (including primary care groups, local health groups and general practices) in England and Wales on a rolling programme every 4 years to undertake a clinical governance review. This will identify best practice to be shared with the rest of the NHS, as well as areas for improvement. A review has three stages – preparation, visit and report – and takes about 26 weeks. The review teams include an NHS doctor or general practitioner, nurse, pharmacist or therapist and a manager.

CHI also investigates serious service failures in the NHS when requested by the Secretary of State for Health in England and the National Assembly for Wales. The Scottish equivalent of CHI is CSBS (Clinical Standards Board for Scotland).

IMPROVING QUALITY IN THE NHS

There are three elements to the government's strategy for improving quality in the NHS (Fig. 7.1):

1. *Set clear national quality standards* – through NSF and NICE or SIGN
2. *Ensure local delivery of high quality clinical services* – through clinical governance, continued professional development (CPD; to ensure that healthcare professional knowledge is contemporary) and professional self-regulation and revalidation (to monitor healthcare professional performance)
3. *Monitor delivery of quality stndards* – through CHI or CSBS, an NHS performance assessment framework (NPAF; not Scotland) and a national survey of patients.

Clinical governance is central to the strategy and has been defined as:

A system through which NHS organizations are accountable for continuously improving the quality of their services and safeguarding high standards of care by creating an

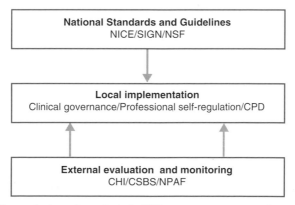

National Standards and Guidelines
NICE/SIGN/NSF

Local implementation
Clinical governance/Professional self-regulation/CPD

External evaluation and monitoring
CHI/CSBS/NPAF

Fig. 7.1 Elements for improving quality in the NHS

environment in which excellence in clinical care will flourish.

Seally & Donaldson 1998[3]

The four main components were set out in the consultation document *A First Class Service: Quality in the new NHS:*[4]

1. *Clear lines of responsibility and accountability for the overall quality of clinical care* – ultimately the Chief Executive of the Trust is responsible but a designated senior clinician should ensure that systems for clinical governance are in place and that they are being monitored

2. *A comprehensive programme of quality improvement activities* – these include: clinical audit; participation in national confidential inquiries; implementation of NICE guidelines; staff training and CPD; safeguarding of information and record storage; research and development

3. *Clear policies aimed at managing risk*

4. *Procedures to identify and remedy poor performance* – these include: incident reporting; complaints procedures; peer review and disciplinary procedures.

The aim of clinical governance is to develop an open learning culture that shares information and makes changes that will improve the quality of care such that there are consistently better outcomes for the patients. This also involves primary care groups, including dentists, pharmacists, district nurses and opticians for whom their relative isolation can make the process very difficult. A clinical governance support team (CGST) has been set up to train and support NHS organizations and their staff in the development of clinical governance systems. A crucial component is *risk management,* i.e. the ability to detect, analyse and learn from events such as adverse incidents and systems failures.

WHAT IS RISK MANAGEMENT?

Risk management (RM) can be defined as a proactive approach which:

1. *addresses* the various activities of an organization
2. *identifies* the risks that exist
3. *assesses* those risks for potential frequency and severity
4. *eliminates* the risks that can be eliminated

5. *reduces* the effect of those that cannot be eliminated
6. *establishes* financial mechanisms to absorb the financial consequence of the risks that remain.

The key aim is to reduce the cost of risk.

PRINCIPLES OF RISK MANAGEMENT

IDENTIFICATION OF RISK

In order to manage a potential risk, it must first be identified. In other words:

- What is the risk?
- How could it occur?
- What is the likely effect of the risk if it is not correctly managed?

Examples of non-clinical risks would be physical hazards such as the storage of dangerous gases or working practices such as inadequate training on lifting patients. A clinical adverse incident occurs when a patient is unintentionally harmed by medical treatment, for example drug errors, awareness while under anaesthetic and unexpected deaths or complications.

ANALYSIS

Once the risk has been identified, it must then be analysed. The questions that must now be asked are:

- How often is the risk likely to occur?
- How much is it likely to cost – both to manage and if it is not controlled?
- What are the potential effects of both the efforts to manage the risk and the likely consequence if the risk is ignored?

There are many different methods of risk identification and analysis, including questionnaires, historical analysis, checklists and physical inspection.

CONTROL

The next step is to consider the measures that must be taken in order to control the risk. It may be possible to eliminate the risk totally or at least avoid it, but it may only be feasible to make it either less likely to occur or cheaper to deal with the outcomes. Examples of such measures include physical controls, such as controlled drugs cupboards or restricted-access areas, as well as, for example, training programmes on lifting or handling hazardous materials.

FUNDING

Funding for RM is part of every hospital budget. Funding for claims in England comes from the Clinical Negligence Scheme for Trusts (CNST) and the Existing Liabilities Scheme (ELS). There are different arrangements for Wales, Scotland and Northern Ireland as detailed below.

86

CLINICAL GOVERNANCE AND RISK MANAGEMENT
► WHY DO WE NEED RISK MANAGEMENT?

WHY DO WE NEED RISK MANAGEMENT?

ALTRUISM

The majority of healthcare
professionals feel a personal and
professional responsibility to
provide patients with the highest
possible standard of care and expect
to work in a safe environment in an
industry with the same aims.

LEGISLATION

Trusts must comply with legislation
such as the *Health and Safety at Work
Act 1974*. Failure to do so can result
in fines, injunctions and the
prosecution of individual managers.

LITIGATION

Both patients and staff are now far
more inclined to take legal action
and to seek compensation than in
the past. Changes in the regulations
on legal aid mean that the
entitlement of a minor to legal aid is
no longer based on the parents'
finances so there are now more
claims for birth injuries. Individual
Trusts are now responsible for the

financial consequences of successful
litigation, leaving less money for
patient care – and this led to the
creation of the CNST.

Trusts are also vicariously
responsible for acts of negligence by
their staff following the introduction
of Crown Indemnity in 1990 and
must meet any resultant claims,
settlement and indirect expenses.
Healthcare professionals are no
longer obliged to be members of a
defence organization.

MEDIA PRESSURE

Incidents such as the Bristol Inquiry
into the Paediatric Cardiac Surgical
service and the Cleveland Inquiry,
where children were allegedly
misdiagnosed as being sexually
abused by their parents, cause
headline news and shake the
public's faith in healthcare
professionals. It is therefore vital to
show that there are systems in place
for the early detection of any future
problems and for a rapid response to
any questions raised.

CNST

The Clinical Negligence Scheme for
Trusts (CNST) was designed and
implemented in April 1995 by the
Medical Protection Society, with
funding from the Department of
Health. It was established under

Section 21 of the *NHS and
Community Care Act 1990* and is
therefore administered by the
Secretary of State through the
National Health Services Litigation
Authority (NHSLA). However, it is

owned by the members who determine its policies and monitor the performance of the contracted managers.

Membership is voluntary but now almost all NHS Trusts are members. It is basically a 'pay as you go' insurance scheme against large negligence costs, i.e. only sufficient money is collected each year to pay out expected claims falling due that year. Excesses are used to offset contributions the following year or refunded to members. Trusts choose their own excess for each claim; this ranges between £20 000 and £250 000. The Trust pays 100% of claims settled below that excess; 20% of claims settled between the excess and an ultimate threshold and the CNST pays 100% of claims above. Cover is on a 'claims paid' basis, i.e. the Trust must be a member at the time of the incident, the time that the claim is made and the time that the claim is settled; legal defence costs are included. Cases arising before 1 April 1995 are dealt with by the Existing Liabilities Scheme, which is managed directly by the NHSLA.

Contributions are now set according to the level of claims made against individual Trusts and are adjusted for risk management and claims handling expertise, turnover and activity. This led to the development of minimum objective standards of RM for each activity category of Trusts which, when achieved, allow the Trust to be considered for a contribution discount. This meant that clinical incident reporting and the development of RM was no longer an optional extra for Trusts. The risk management programme is managed on behalf of the NHSLA by Willis Corroon, Bristol.

RM STANDARDS

The aims of the RM standards are that they should:

- be measurable and achievable
- improve patient care
- raise awareness of RM
- improve standards and procedures
- reduce the level of claims
- reflect risk exposure
- ensure that the member's contributions to the CNST reflect their standards of RM.

There are 10 'core' standards, plus 'Standard 11' (see below). The latter deals specifically with maternity care and is the only clinical standard that has yet to be developed. The standards are then further subdivided into three levels of achievement that are designed to reflect the degree of difficulty in attaining that level. The aim is to assist Trusts in developing their risk strategy over time and to reward those that comply.

There is a compulsory visit from a CNST assessor in the first year and the Trust is scored on the achievement of level 1 standards.

The RM standards

1. The Board has a written RM policy that makes their commitment to RM explicit
2. An Executive Director of the Board is charged with the responsibility for RM throughout the Trust
3. The responsibility for the management and coordination of clinical risk is clear
4. A clinical incident reporting system is operated in all medical specialties and clinical support departments
5. There is a policy for the rapid follow-up of major clinical incidents
6. An agreed system of managing complaints is in place
7. Appropriate information is provided to patients on the risks and benefits of the proposed treatment or investigation, and the alternatives available, before a signature on a consent form is sought
8. A comprehensive system for the completion, use, storage and retrieval of medical records is in place. Record-keeping standards are monitored through the clinical audit process
9. There is an induction or orientation programme for all new staff
10. A RM system is in place
11. There is a clear documented system for management and communication throughout the key stages of maternity care

The onus is on the Trust to prove that it has achieved the standard through policy documents, development of clinical guidelines, etc. and the discount in contributions depends on that score. Further discounts apply as the Trust attains levels 2 and 3. The Trust can apply for reassessment at any time it feels that it has satisfied the criteria for the next level, but only once per year. There are then random visits in subsequent years to ensure that the Trust is adhering to the standards.

FUNDING FOR CLAIMS IN WALES

Trusts in Wales can join the All Wales Risk Pool, which is managed by the Welsh Office and covers both clinical and non-clinical risks. The excess varies with each individual case and the premium paid by each Trust is a percentage of the Trust budget. The Pool has a set of RM standards similar to those of the CNST but they are not exactly the same and are managed by the District Audit. The Welsh Office also provides legal support through a common services agency.

FUNDING FOR CLAIMS IN SCOTLAND AND NORTHERN IRELAND

The situation in Scotland and Northern Ireland is essentially the same as when Crown Indemnity was introduced in 1990.

The level of litigation in Scotland is very low and the Scottish Central Legal Office acts for the Trusts. Claims are paid out of the Scottish Pool and there are no set RM standards.

The level of litigation in Northern Ireland is much higher and claims are paid out of a Common Fund. There are no RM standards and the Trusts obtain their legal advice from a list of approved solicitors.

CLAIMS HANDLING

Both the CNST and the ELS rely upon their members reporting claims directly to them using a specific report form. Trusts must also update their information on any outstanding claims every 3 months.

Claims from the CNST are categorized as follows:

- *Category A claims* – claims that fall below a Trust's chosen excess and must be reported once the claim is closed
- *Category B claims* – claims that fall above the chosen excess but below £500 000
- *Category C claims* – claims where the settlement is above £500 000.

Both category B and C claims must be reported as soon the initial request for compensation has been made and the value assessed.

Claims handled by the ELS are inevitably older so the process is more complicated. Trusts must submit a detailed 7-page report form and a full set of disclosures, including expert witness reports.

Once the formal report form has been submitted, the relevant claims manager or solicitors acting for the NHSLA liaise with the local claims manager or trust solicitor in order to assess:

- the merits of the case (this includes a review of any documentation, witnesses and experts)
- the litigation risks
- the economics of the case
- any 'audit trail' to justify any recommendations.

LIABILITIES

Some 80% of liabilities arise from 20% of claims, with 60% arising from just 3% of claims. Obstetric cases provide for 70% of the CNST's current contingent liability by *value* although the actual *number* of claims is more evenly spread throughout the specialties.

An important type of liability is the 'incurred but not reported' (IBNR) liability, i.e. an incident has occurred that is likely to cost the Trust or the CNST money but it has either not yet been reported or paid. For example:

1. 1996 – a patient is harmed as a result of negligence by the Trust.

2. 1998 – the patient becomes aware that his injury occurred as a result of negligence, reports the injury and the case is investigated.

3. 2000 – the Trust is found negligent.

4. 2001 – the patient is paid compensation.

5. A proportion of the Trust budget for 2001 must now be used to settle a claim for an injury that occurred in 1996 unless it is paid by the CNST.

6. In order for the CNST to settle the claim in full, the Trust must have been a member from 1996 to 2001 and the claim must be above £500 000.

INCIDENT REPORTING

Most Trusts use one incident form for all adverse incidents, regardless of origin, but some separate clinical incidents from non-clinical. Some allow staff to use other avenues such as the telephone or e-mail and accept anonymous reporting. While the latter may be essential for incident reporting to be a blame-free process, it can make it very difficult to fully investigate an incident.

Most Trusts also give their staff training in incident reporting – both in the actual process and what constitutes an adverse incident but there is little standardization between Trusts over what is considered to be an adverse event.

Adverse incidents are common and they are only rarely the result of a single failure in the process, such as one individual. The surgeon may be criticized when an operation goes wrong, but it may be that he was using inadequate equipment or had insufficient light. It has been shown that adverse conditions such as high workload, inadequate supervision or poor communication increase liability to error.[5] Investigations that consider only the acts of individual healthcare professionals are therefore inadequate and may be misleading. They also serve to discourage future reporting.

Incident data should be subjected

to analysis, both at a local individual and on a corporate aggregate basis, in order to reap the most benefit from it. It is particularly important to document near misses and to identify common themes in order to predict and prevent future incidents.

The effectiveness of incident reporting can be measured in three ways:

1. The number of changes in practice that have resulted from it
2. Its success in alerting the Trust to potential complaints and/or litigation
3. The amount of feedback given to clinicians.

In order for a reporting scheme to be effective it must:

- be mandatory
- be confidential
- foster a blame-free culture of learning and enquiring to encourage reporting
- provide information about general organizational failures as well as specific events
- categorize serious adverse events and research them to identify trigger factors
- have a system for analysing and disseminating information and lessons from incidents and near misses
- implement the important lessons and make any necessary changes
- provide support and feedback to the staff involved to give positive reinforcement.

References
1. Department of Health. The New NHS: modern, dependable. London: DoH, 1997
2. Ellis S. Some unanswered questions about NICE. J R Soc Med 1998; 91: 538–539
3. Scally G, Donaldson L. Clinical governance and the drive for quality improvement in the new NHS in England. BMJ 1998; 317: 1725–1727
4. Department of Health. A first class service: quality in the new NHS. London: DoH, 1998
5. Vincent C, Taylor-Adams S, Stanhope N. Framework for analysing risk and safety in clinical medicine. BMJ 1998; 316: 1154–1157

Further reading
CNST. Risk management standards and procedures: manual of guidance © NHSLA Willis Corroon Ltd, Bristol, 1997
NHS Executive. Clinical governance; quality in the new NHS. London: DoH, 1999

Useful websites
CGST: www.cgsupport.org
CHI: www.chi.nhs.uk
Clinical Governance Bulletin: www.clinical-governance.com
NICE: www.nice.org.uk

CHAPTER 8

HANDLING COMPLAINTS

INTRODUCTION

In 1996, a new NHS complaints procedure was introduced that replaced the previously separate ones for family practitioners (general dental and medical practitioners, pharmacists and opticians) and for hospital and community services. It also separated the complaint from any disciplinary procedure. It has since been adapted and is now based on the seven core principles of accessibility, simplicity, speed, fairness, confidentiality, effectiveness and quality enhancement as set out in the Wilson Committee report, *Being Heard*.[1] It was designed to give a quick, informal response at a local level, but allowed the complainant the opportunity to ask for an independent review panel if he was not satisfied with the reply. There was also a third level if he was still not satisfied, this being the Health Service Ombudsman with new powers to investigate clinical complaints.

WHY PATIENTS COMPLAIN

In 1999–2000, there were nearly 40 000 written complaints about family health services and over 86 500 about hospital and community health services, including ambulance trusts. The number continues to rise but it seems to relate to changes in patient expectations and acceptance as there is no evidence to suggest that the number of mistakes made by healthcare professionals has risen. Note that the Patient's Charter actively encourages patients to complain if they are dissatisfied, theoretically to improve the service, and advises them of their 'right' to an investigation and a written reply.

The commonest sources of complaint are:

● 'all aspects of treatment'
● staff attitudes
● delays and cancellation of outpatient appointments
● missed or incorrect diagnosis.

The reasons that patients give for bringing the complaint include:

● acknowledgement that there has been a problem
● wanting answers or an apology
● needing assurance that what has happened to them or to a relative will not happen to others
● wanting to know what remedial actions, if any, will be taken to prevent such an event happening again
● wanting financial compensation
● wanting the member(s) of staff involved to be punished.

For a complaint to be investigated under the complaints procedure, it must originate within 6 months of the event or within

6 months of the complainant becoming aware of cause for complaint, although this must not be more than a year since the event. This time limit can be extended at the discretion of the Health Service Ombudsman if there are mitigating circumstances.

The three stages to the complaints procedure comprise: local resolution, independent review and the Health Service Ombudsman.

STAGE 1: LOCAL RESOLUTION

Both hospitals and family health practitioners must have complaints procedures in operation that are approved by the health authority and the local medical committee. All Trusts and practices should publicize their complaints procedures to both staff and patients and provide explanatory leaflets. Records of complaints should be kept separately from the patient's notes and both Trusts and practices must provide the health authority with data relating to the number and type of complaints received. Hospitals must have one or more designated complaints managers and general practices must appoint a member of staff whose specific role is to deal with complaints. This is often the practice manager and this may be a source of conflict, particularly where the manager is an employee of the person being complained about.

The complaint should be investigated by the complaints manager on behalf of either the Chief Executive or the senior principal of the practice, in accordance with the time-scale outlined in Table 8.1.

Note that if it is not possible to meet these targets, the complainant must be kept fully informed of the delay and the underlying reasons. The emphasis is on the rapid, and preferably informal, resolution of complaints. Members of staff are

TABLE 8.1 Response times for events relating to local resolution of complaints

Event	Time allowed
Oral complaint	Dealt with immediately or referred
Acknowledgement of written complaints	Within 2 working days of receipt or full reply within 5 working days
Full response by Trust or health authority	Within 20 working days of receipt
Full response by family health services practitioner	Within 10 working days of receipt for practice-based complaints
Application by complainant for independent review	Within 28 calendar days of receipt of response to local resolution

encouraged to deal with complaints as they arise but they should refer any that they feel warrant further investigation or when they do not feel they can give adequate reassurance to the complainant. All complaints should receive a full written response from either the Chief Executive or the senior principal, aimed at satisfying the complainant and providing an apology and/or explanation where appropriate. Responses to complaints regarding medical care must be agreed with the healthcare professional(s) involved.

If the complainant is dissatisfied with the response, then further attempts can be made at conciliation, including meetings with the healthcare professional(s) involved. If this is unsuccessful then the complainant can request an independent review, either orally or in writing. Note that this is not an automatic right and will not be recommended if litigation is pending.

STAGE 2: INDEPENDENT REVIEW

Of all complainants to hospitals last year, 2.4% requested an independent review, of which about 10% were referred for a panel. For practice-based complaints, 3.5% requested an independent review and nearly 25% were referred. Requests for an independent review are considered by the convenor, who is a non-executive director of the Trust or health authority. Note that this has led to allegations that this makes the system biased against the complainant and it may be difficult for the convenor to maintain his independence.

The role of the convenor is to:

1. obtain a statement from the complainant, which sets out his remaining grievances
2. ensure an impartial view
3. check that all avenues have already been explored in order to settle the complaint at a local level

4. decide whether or not an independent review panel should be established and what its terms of reference should be. This decision should only be made after consultation with the lay chairman and, if the complaint relates to clinical judgement, after obtaining independent clinical advice.

The convenor must adhere to the targets shown in Table 8.2.

The independent review panel consists of three members:

1. an independent lay chairman nominated by the Secretary of State from a regional list
2. the convenor
3. a representative of the Trust, general practice or health authority.

If the complaint relates to exercise of clinical judgement, then the panel is advised by at least two

TABLE 8.2 Response times for events relating to independent review of complaints

Event	Time allowed
Acknowledgement by convenor for independent review	Within 2 working days of receipt
Decision by convenor whether or not to set up panel	Within 20 working days of receipt (10 for practice-based complaints)
Appointment of panel members	Within 20 working days of decision (10 for practice-based complaints)
Draft report of panel	Within 50 working days of formal appointment of panel (30 for practice-based complaints)
Final report of panel	Within 10 further working days
Response to complainant	Within 20 days of receipt of panel's report (5 for practice-based complaints)

independent clinical assessors, nominated by the regional office. There must be at least one assessor for each specialty and profession involved and their reports must be attached to the final report of the panel.

A panel will not be set up where:

- there is legal action pending
- the trust, health authority or general practice has already taken all practicable action
- there is further action still possible at the local resolution stage.

If the convenor makes the decision not to set up a panel, then the complainant must be informed and advised of the reasons. They should also be advised of their right to take the complaint to the Health Service Ombudsman.

The panel investigates the aspects of the complaint that are set out in its terms of reference and makes a report setting out its conclusions and recommendations. The proceedings must be confidential and the panel must have access to all the relevant documentation. The complainant and those complained about must be given an opportunity to express their opinions but they cannot be legally represented. The panel has no authority over any subsequent actions by the Trust, health authority or family practitioner and it cannot recommend any disciplinary action. Copies of the report are sent to the complainant, the clinical assessors, the Trust or health authority chairman and the chief executive or practitioner concerned. The chief executive or senior partner of the practice should then write to the complainant within 4 weeks, informing him of any remedial action to be taken and his right to take his complaint to the Ombudsman if he is still not satisfied.

STAGE 3: THE HEALTH SERVICE OMBUDSMAN

The Health Service Commissioner or Ombudsman provides an independent investigation of complaints about services under the NHS. It is a Crown appointment and the office is entirely independent of both the government and the NHS. The powers and jurisdiction of the office are governed by the *Health Service Commissioners Act 1993*, which was amended in 1996 to allow the Ombudsman to investigate complaints related to clinical judgement. The complainant must be the aggrieved party, his personal representative or a family member. It cannot be a public authority. The complaint must be in writing and the incident should have occurred within the past year unless there are mitigating factors. The Ombudsman has the same rights of access to persons and documents as the High Court but the investigations must be done in private.

The Ombudsman can, at his discretion, investigate complaints of hardship or injustice as a consequence of:

● failure in a service provided by a health service body
● failure of such a body to provide a service
● maladministration connected with any other action taken on behalf of such a body
● clinical complaints following events arising on or after 1 April 1996.

Examples of such complaints include waiting lists, poor communication, cancellation of operations, confidentiality issues and handling of complaints.

The Ombudsman cannot investigate complaints:

● that have not been through the NHS complaints procedure
● where an appeal is possible
● where litigation is in process
● where the primary concern is financial compensation
● where the patient has a remedy in a court or before a tribunal, unless the Ombudsman believes that it would be unreasonable to expect the complainant to take that option
● relating to NHS contracts – either with staff or with other bodies, e.g. cleaning.

Clinical complaints are reviewed by medical advisers to the Ombudsman. If they consider that the management is not open to criticism, then the Ombudsman will advise the complainant that there will be no intervention, giving the reasons for doing so. If there are grounds for questioning the clinical judgement, then the case will be investigated using external professional assessors from the relevant specialty. The investigation may be based solely on the notes but can involve interviews with the relevant staff. The investigators then produce a report of their findings, which takes the form of a peer review, using the 'Bolam' standard (see Ch. 9). The Ombudsman then reports in confidence to the complainant, with copies to the Secretary of State and the body against which the complaint was made.

If the Ombudsman finds that there has been a deficiency in the actions of either an individual practitioner or a NHS body, then he will ask them to agree to an apology being conveyed to the complainant in the report. If he considers that remedial action is required, then he will recommend it but he has no power to force either an apology or remedial action. However, if the practitioner or the NHS body refuses to accept the recommendations, then they may have to appear before the Select Committee of the House of Commons, which oversees the work of the Ombudsman. After the report has been made, the NHS body or the practitioner must inform the Ombudsman within 3 months of any actions taken to implement the recommendations. There is no appeal procedure if either party is dissatisfied with the report – the only redress available is a judicial review, but there has yet to be a test case.

RESPONDING TO A COMPLAINT

When asked to respond to a complaint, always consider the following:

- Investigate the complaint thoroughly. This should include interviews with all the staff involved and taking statements where necessary. You should also perform a comprehensive review of the notes and assess the situation at the time of the complaint. For example, if the complaint involves an attendance at the Accident & Emergency department, then you should consider the staffing levels, waiting times, number of attendances and the case mix.
- Be prompt in your reply – bear in mind the time limits.

- Include an expression of regret that the complainant was unhappy with the service provided.
- Apologize where it is appropriate but do not try to defend situations beyond your control, e.g. inadequate staffing levels.
- Describe in detail the circumstances that contributed to the complaint, e.g. waiting times.
- If other parties are also involved, ensure that you have received a report from them and that they are aware that you are replying to the complaint on their behalf.
- Provide a factual reply that specifically addresses *all* the points made in the complaint, preferably enumerating each point.

- **Never** be defensive or appear hostile towards the complainant.
- If practice has changed as a result of the complaint in an effort to prevent a recurrence, then tell the complainant as this may be all they wanted.
- Be aware of the possibility that the complaint is simply an exercise in gathering information for future litigation.
- Complaints are often an opportunity to remind the management that there are deficiencies in the service provided that need to be addressed, such as inadequate facilities or supervision of junior staff.

Reference
1. Department of Health. Being heard. The report of a review committee on NHS complaints procedures. London: DoH, 1999

Further reading
Department of Health. Handling complaints: monitoring the NHS complaints procedures. London: DoH, 2000
NHS Executive. Complaints – listening … acting … improving: guidance on the implementation of the NHS complaints procedure. London: DoH, 1994

Useful websites
Department of Health:
www.open.gov.uk/doh
Health Service Commissioner:
www.ombudsman.org.uk

CHAPTER 9

CLINICAL NEGLIGENCE

DEFINITION OF CLINICAL NEGLIGENCE

In the UK, unless the negligence has been so gross as to amount to a criminal act, most cases of alleged clinical negligence are regarded as *torts* or civil wrongs and are dealt with through civil proceedings.

For an allegation of negligence by a healthcare professional to succeed, the claimant must prove all four of the following:

1. The defendant had a *duty of care* to the claimant
2. There was a *breach* of that duty of care
3. The claimant suffered *actionable harm or damage*
4. The damage was caused by the breach *(causation).*

DUTY OF CARE

All healthcare professionals have a duty to become and remain competent at their job and they should be diligent in providing those skills to those that have need of them. The various professional bodies, such as the General Medical Council (GMC) or the Nursing and Midwifery Council (NMC) (see Ch. 10), set the minimum standards necessary, but the level of skill and proficiency will vary with experience, continuing education and seniority. If a senior healthcare professional delegates a task to a more junior one, he must be confident that his colleague has sufficient experience and skill to do it since he still carries part, if not all, responsibility for any resultant errors. This is known as *vicarious liability* and also applies to Trusts, who are held to be legally responsible for the actions of the staff that they employ. Vicarious liability does *not* apply to allegations arising from 'Good Samaritan' acts

or other activities (e.g. the provision of statements or private medical reports) so all healthcare professionals should have private insurance or belong to a defence society. General practitioners are vicariously responsible for the staff that they employ (e.g. receptionists or nurses), but *not* for locums or deputizing doctors. They are also responsible for any claims made against them so *must* have private insurance or belong to a defence society.

In some cases, it is obvious that the healthcare professional owes a duty of care, for example a patient with a 'named nurse' or those who are on the practice list or have paid a fee for a service. However, a duty of care can be legally shown in other situations, such as a doctor stopping at a roadside to offer assistance following a car crash. In some countries, doctors are legally required to stop at the site of a car accident and can be prosecuted if it can be proved that they drove past. In the UK, however, 'Good Samaritan' acts remain an ethical duty only.

If a healthcare professional examines a patient for any purpose other than to provide advice or treatment, there is no established duty of care (e.g. insurance, drink-drive or pre-employment examinations). If the patient is harmed during the examination, then he is entitled to sue the healthcare professional but he cannot accuse him of negligence if he is refused insurance on the basis of the medical report. In such cases, the duty of the healthcare professional is to the insurance company, not the patient.

BREACH OF DUTY OF CARE

A healthcare professional breaches his duty of care if he fails to reach the level of proficiency of his peers. This is known as the *Bolam test* and it applies equally to the duty to treat, diagnose and give advice. It follows the case of *Bolam v Friern Hospital Management Committee 1957*,[1] where the claimant was given electroconvulsive therapy without sedation or manual restraint and suffered bilateral hip fractures as a result. He sued the hospital for negligence but the claim was dismissed on the basis that his management was the standard practice at that time. The judge, Mr Justice McNair, said that a doctor was not negligent if he acted in accordance with a responsible and competent body of relevant professional opinion even if other doctors adopted a different practice. It is important to remember that courts maintain the right to decide whether an established medical practice is acceptable or not so it may not be sufficient to provide expert opinion to support a particular treatment. It is also important to note that, in Scotland, the test case was that of *Hunter v Hanley*[2] and the ruling stated that a doctor had to act in accordance with a 'responsible doctor' so the standard is potentially lower.

Ignorance is no defence in negligence and the case of *Wilsher v Essex Area Health Authority*[3] ruled that the duty of care of a junior healthcare professional includes an obligation to seek senior advice. Although a junior cannot be expected to have the same skills as a senior, the duty of care relates to the act and patients are entitled to optimum care, independent of the provider. If a junior does not have the skill or experience to proficiently perform a procedure, then he *must* defer to his senior.

Note that genuine errors of clinical judgement are not the same as negligence. All healthcare professionals make mistakes but if they can show that they exercised reasonable skill and care in coming to their decision, then they cannot be held to have been negligent even if that decision was wrong (e.g. an incorrect diagnosis or treatment).

The breach can be something:

- done (commission), e.g. forceps left in the chest after heart surgery
- not done (omission), e.g. failure to attend a sick patient.

ACTIONABLE HARM OR DAMAGE

This is the disability, loss or injury suffered by the claimant and it is distinct from 'damages', which is the financial compensation awarded to a successful claimant. However negligent the defendant has been, the claimant must have suffered quantifiable harm as a result in order for the action to be successful, for example if a doctor delays in diagnosing a particular condition, then he is only negligent if the delay adversely affects the final outcome. *Quantifiable harm* includes: loss of earnings; reduced quality or quantity of life; disfigurement; disability and mental anguish.

There may also be an element of *contributory negligence,* where the actions of the claimant are judged to have made the situation worse (e.g. removing a dressing or failing to attend follow-up appointments). This does not affect the judgment but can reduce the amount of damages awarded. If the claimant was off work as a result of the injury and received social security benefits such as statutory sick pay, then under the *Social Security Administration Act 1992,* an amount equal to the benefits will be subtracted from the compensation payment. The corresponding provision in Northern Ireland is the *Social Security Administration (Northern Ireland) Act 1992.* These Acts apply to injuries or diseases that occurred after 1 January 1989 and the deduction is paid directly to the Department of Social Security by the compensator. If the injury occurred before 1 January 1989, then the compensator keeps the deduction. There are some exemptions such as payments of £2500 or less, those made under the *Vaccine Damage Payments Act 1979* or those from the Criminal Injuries Compensation Board.

CAUSATION

Causation is the link between the actionable harm and the breach of duty of care, i.e. on a balance of probabilities, it is more likely that the harm suffered by the claimant resulted from the actions of the defendant.

THE LEGAL PROCESS

The burden of proof is on the claimant, i.e. he must prove that the defendant has been negligent and the standard of proof is the civil standard – the *balance of probabilities* (see Ch. 2). The only exceptions are cases where the facts are so obvious that the onus is on the healthcare professional to prove that he was not negligent (e.g. amputation of the wrong foot). This is the doctrine of *res ipsa loquitur* ('the facts speak for themselves') but these almost invariably settle out of court.

Under the *Limitation Act 1980,* actions for negligence must be brought within 3 years of the *date of knowledge,* which is either the date on which the alleged negligence occurred or when the patient became aware of the effects, which may be years later. There are exceptions to this rule: if the claimant was a child at the time of the injury, the limitation period starts at 18 and if he was mentally ill, it starts at the date of recovery. The court can also allow cases out of time to proceed if it would not prejudice either party to do so – one recent case was settled for £1.25m 33 years after the original damage to his brain that occurred during birth. This means that it is often very difficult to defend negligence cases and emphasizes the importance of making good contemporaneous notes.

Following the introduction of the new Civil Procedure Rules, both parties must follow the preaction protocol developed by the Clinical Disputes Forum. This has a *commitments* section, which sets out the principles that both the healthcare provider and the patient should follow. For the healthcare provider, these are essentially the same as those for clinical risk management (see Ch. 7), while the patient has an obligation to bring any concerns to the attention of the healthcare provider as early as possible. He must also consider all the options available, including negotiation and the complaints procedures (see Ch. 8) before starting litigation. The steps section (Fig. 9.1) sets out a recommended sequence of actions to be followed if litigation is in prospect.

Explanation for Figure 9.1

a. The Letter of Claim informs the recipient of the dates of the alleged negligent treatment and the events giving rise to the claim. It also details the injuries, condition and future prognosis, with an outline of the causal link between the injuries and the allegations. It may also include a request for the medical notes if they have not already been provided, as well as the likely value of the claim. It may also include an offer to settle. The defendant must acknowledge the Letter of Claim within 14 days and provide copies of the requested records within 40 days.

b. The Letter of Response must be provided within 3 months and should comment on the events if

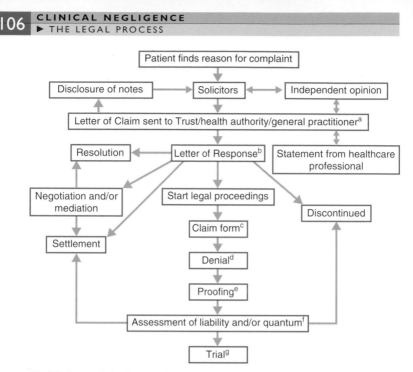

Fig. 9.1 Steps in the legal process following a complaint (see text for explanation of symbols a–g)

they are disputed, with details of any other documentation upon which the defendant intends to rely. If breach of duty and causation are accepted, then suggestions may be made regarding resolution and/or settlement.

c. Civil courts now issue claim forms instead of writs or originating summons. They contain particulars of the alleged negligence and resultant harm.

d. Following the introduction of the Civil Procedure Rules, the defendant must now specify the reasons for any denial and state his own version of events if it differs from that of the claimant.

e. 'Proofing' means that the defendant's solicitors prepare answers to the particulars.

f. Assessment of quantum means that the level of financial compensation is estimated based on previous settlements for similar injuries and standard textbooks. If it is likely to cost more to defend the case than to settle, the defendant may consider this to be the better option although there is then an implication of guilt that will then not be contested. If the Trust is defending the action and decides to settle, the healthcare professional(s) involved will probably not be consulted and may be left feeling that justice has not been served. Assessment of liability means that all the evidence is considered. If it appears that the defendant is liable, then the case is settled.

g. Only about 5% of cases go to court and are decided by the judge on the basis of expert opinion.

LEGAL AID

Legal aid is designed to allow access to justice for those who cannot afford legal services. However, under the current system, most people are ineligible, so only the very rich or the very poor can afford to bring a legal action. The Legal Services Commission grants legal aid but it depends on advice from the applicant's solicitor, who may make the case appear more meritorious than it actually is in order to obtain funding. It has been retained for medical negligence cases but abolished for other types of personal injury claim following the introduction of the conditional fee scheme in 1995, which allows solicitors to accept cases on a 'no win, no fee' basis.

Legal aid also includes a costs protection in that if a legally aided person loses his case, he does not have to pay the winner's legal costs, making the system inherently unfair. There are thus more speculative legally aided cases and there is less incentive for them to settle out of court. In medical negligence cases, Trusts will often settle legally aided cases simply to avoid irrecoverable legal costs.

NO-FAULT COMPENSATION

In some countries, such as Sweden and New Zealand, the claimant need only show that the injury resulted from 'medical or surgical misadventure' and compensation is based on need. The claimant does not have to prove negligence by the healthcare professional involved. However, if the injury followed a complication, then it may be difficult to show that it was so rare as to constitute a misadventure, i.e. not avoidable through the exercise of reasonable care. It is also often hard to distinguish between a consequence of treatment and of the natural progress of the disease. Note that in New Zealand, *all* medical error findings are referred for consideration of disciplinary or criminal proceedings so it is a very hostile environment in which to practise medicine.

THE FUTURE

In 1994, Lord Woolf was appointed to inquire into the civil justice system of England and Wales. In his final report[4] he stated that the existing system for dealing with medical negligence actions was failing both claimants and defendants in the following respects:

1. There was a disproportionate relationship between costs and the amount awarded, particularly in low-value cases.
2. The delay before claims were settled was longer for medical negligence cases than for any other type of civil action.
3. Unmeritorious cases were pursued and clear-cut cases defended for longer than for any other type of civil action.
4. The success rate was lower than any other personal injury litigation.
5. There was less cooperation and more animosity between the opposing parties than in other classes of litigation, with experts becoming partisan advocates, rather than neutral givers of opinion.

He also found that over 90% of litigants were legally aided, as were 92% of the successful litigants. As those that are eligible for legal aid are not more vulnerable to negligence than those who are not, then it is likely that a change in the provision of financial assistance would bring a greater number of more successful actions.

Lord Woolf's proposals for change included:

● case management by the courts to allow better throughput of cases and improved access by encouraging cooperation between the parties and, if possible, settlement
● alternative dispute resolution, including mediation (see Ch. 4)
● court-based experts or a single expert approved by both parties to provide a report
● Judges with specialist medical knowledge.

The report also led to the development of the new Civil Procedure Rules 1998, which replaced both the Rules of the Supreme Court and the County Court Rules, and came into force in April 1999. However, a report from the National Audit Office in May 2001 estimated the cost of settling outstanding and expected claims to be £3.9bn. It also noted that and it still takes an average of $5^1/_2$ years to settle a claim and that for small claims (up to £50 000), the legal costs continue to outweigh the damages in over 65% of cases. This has stimulated the government to find alternatives to the current compensation system and the proposals under consideration are:

● No-fault compensation
● Early settlement using a fixed tariff of payments depending on the injury caused (similar to the Criminal Injuries Compensation scheme)

- More use of structured settlements providing annuities rather than lump sums

- Greater use of mediation to settle disputes.

CRIMINAL NEGLIGENCE

Although more common than previously, criminal convictions for negligence are still very rare and effectively limited to prosecutions for manslaughter. In *R v Bateman*,[5] the judge stressed that for criminal liability to be established, the negligence must go beyond compensation to such disregard for life and safety as to amount to a crime against the State. The most famous case was that of *R v Adomako*,[6] where an anaesthetist failed to recognize that the patient was in distress and there was conflicting evidence to suggest that he was either present and grossly incompetent or not actually in the theatre, having left the patient without adequate monitoring. The patient died and Dr Adomako was convicted of manslaughter. In New Zealand, a healthcare professional can be found criminally liable merely for failing to exercise 'reasonable knowledge, skill and care'!

References

1. *Bolam v Friern Hospital Management Committee* [1957] 2 All ER 118
2. *Hunter v Hanley* [1955] SC 200
3. *Wilsher v Essex Area Health Authority* [1986] 3 All ER 801 (CA); [1988] 1 All ER 871 (HL)
4. Access to justice: final report by the Right Honourable Lord Woolf. London: HMSO, 1996
5. *R v Bateman* [1925] All ER Rep 45 at 48
6. *R v Adomako* [1991] 2 Med LR 277

Useful websites

Action for Victims of Medical Accidents: www.avma.org.uk
Legal information: www.medical-accidents.co.uk

CHAPTER 10

DISCIPLINARY BODIES AND PROCEDURES

INTRODUCTION

Regulation of standards varies enormously between the different healthcare professions from statutory disciplinary proceedings to guidelines set by bodies that also negotiate levels of pay and working conditions. However, the majority of these bodies do set standards to which the healthcare professional must adhere and have disciplinary procedures for those that fail to do so. The concept of 'self-regulation' by the various professional bodies has led to increasing public concern and the structure and function of all three of the councils now described are currently under review with major changes likely in the near future.

THE GENERAL MEDICAL COUNCIL (GMC)

The GMC and the medical register were established by the *Medical Act 1858*. The GMC is an independent statutory body that is responsible for medical registration, regulation, education and discipline in the UK and gains its current powers from the *Medical Act 1983*. There are 104 members, of which 54 are elected, 25 are appointed by educational bodies and 25 are lay members, nominated by the Privy Council. The functions of the GMC are as follows.

THE MEDICAL REGISTER

The GMC maintains the medical register that allows all doctors to be identified for legal and official purposes. It gives the doctor's full name, date of birth, primary and any higher qualifications. In the UK, newly qualified doctors have only provisional registration for the first year, which limits their practice, for example they cannot make the decision to discharge patients. After satisfactory completion of the 'preregistration' year as a house officer, the doctor then becomes fully registered. Other doctors may be eligible for limited or provisional registration and this is determined by both the *Medical Act 1983* and the regulations and decisions of the GMC. Such decisions involve consideration of knowledge of English, specialist skills and the type of qualification. There are four separate lists:

1. *Principal list* – all doctors resident in the UK
2. *Overseas list* – doctors living outside the UK and the European Union (EU)
3. *Visiting overseas doctors list* – doctors who have qualified overseas but have been granted temporary full registration for the provision of specialist services
4. *Visiting EU practitioners list* – similar to (3) but the doctors have qualified in the EU.

EDUCATION

The Education Committee consists of 19 members, including two lay members and a medical student representative. It promotes high standards of education and is responsible for undergraduate and general clinical training. The role includes coordination of all the stages of medical education, curriculum changes and inspection of qualifying examinations from all examining bodies, including the Royal Colleges and medical schools. In 1996, the GMC was required to establish a specialist register under the *European Specialist Medical Qualifications Order 1995*, and inclusion on the list is determined by the Specialist Training Authority. Inclusion depends on the successful completion of either 5 or 6 years of training in a specialty, with annual assessments and, for some specialties, fulfilment of an 'exit' examination.

DISCIPLINARY PROCEDURES

The *Medical Act 1983* created three committees to deal with the responsibilities of the GMC in relation to professional conduct and fitness to practice. These are:

1. *The Preliminary Proceedings Committee (PPC).* This has 12 members – ten medical and two lay.
2. *The Professional Conduct Committee (PCC).* This has 32 members, of which six are lay. Cases are usually heard by 11 members.

3. *The Health Committee (HC).* This has 12 members, of which one is lay.

The GMC received 4470 complaints in 2000, representing a 50% rise on 1999, although 25% did not come within the remit of the GMC. The police are required to notify the GMC if a doctor is convicted of *any* criminal offence and offences involving personal conduct, for example misuse of alcohol or drugs, dishonesty, indecency, fraud or violence. Other sources of complaint include: statutory declarations from patients or relatives; reports from hospital managers; referrals from the Secretary of State; newspaper reports or other doctors. All complaints are referred to a preliminary screener, who is a medical member of the GMC responsible for deciding whether or not the complaint comes within the jurisdiction of the GMC. The screener can refer a case to the PPC alone but he cannot reject it without first discussing it with a lay member. If the case is referred, the GMC writes to the practitioner with details of the allegation and invites a written explanation for submission to the PPC.

The PPC meets in private five times a year and decides, on written evidence only, whether or not to refer the case to the PCC for an oral hearing. This occurs in about a third of all cases but the PPC can also:

- decide to take no action
- write a letter of advice or warning
- suspend or place conditions on registration for up to 2 months

but only if the doctor has been given an opportunity of appearing before the PPC; it is only effective until the doctor is seen by either the PCC or the HC
- refer the doctor to the HC if there is reason to believe that the practitioner is suffering from physical or mental illness that impairs his fitness to practice.

Hearings of the PCC are public and witnesses may be compelled to appear by subpoena. Oral evidence is given on oath and the practitioner is entitled to legal representation. The doctor can dispute and rebut evidence, and misconduct must be *proved by evidence* unless the doctor admits it. If the facts are proved to the criminal standard of *beyond reasonable doubt,* the PCC must decide whether or not it amounts to serious professional misconduct. This includes:

- abuse of professional privileges or skills, e.g. unlawful prescription of controlled drugs or sexual relationships with patients
- conduct derogatory to the reputation of the medical profession, e.g. indecent or violent behaviour, fraud, forgery
- advertising
- disparagement of professional colleagues
- disregard or neglect of professional duties, e.g. inappropriate delegation or failing to provide treatment.

The PCC must also consider testimonials and the past history of the doctor. Note that both the PPC and PCC act as judicial bodies and may be advised by a legal assessor, who is usually a Queen's Counsel of at least 10 years' standing. At the conclusion of the inquiry, the PCC must decide to:

- conclude the case
- refer the doctor to the HC
- postpone determination, in which case the doctor remains on the register but must give the GMC the names of professional colleagues to whom they can apply for information regarding his conduct since the previous hearing. If the information is satisfactory, then the case is usually concluded. If not, then the GMC can:
  — impose restrictions on practice for up to 3 years, for example restrictions on prescriptions of controlled drugs or remedial training (e.g. in clinical skills)
  — suspend the doctor for up to 1 year
  — erase the doctor from the register. This is effective unless and until the doctor makes a successful application for restoration which must be at least 10 months after the erasure. If the application is unsuccessful, then the doctor must wait a further 10 months before reapplying.

Doctors have the right of appeal within 28 days to the Judicial Committee of the Privy Council. The practitioner continues on the register until appeal if it is granted unless the PCC has made an order for immediate suspension.

If a doctor is convicted in the UK

of a criminal offence, even if it is not related to his professional conduct, then he can:

- be erased from register
- have his registration suspended for not more than 1 year
- have conditions attached to his registration for up to 3 years.

Currently, the GMC acts as judge, jury and prosecutor, but proposed reforms to the GMC[1] strongly support the separation of judgement and prosecution, making the process much more robust, transparent and fair.

THE 'SICK' DOCTOR

The GMC has statutory procedures to deal with practitioners referred because of health problems, the majority being alcohol or drug-related or due to mental illness. The procedure is confidential and has four stages:

1. The preliminary screener considers the complaint, often from a concerned colleague. If he identifies a possible impairment of fitness:
2. The doctor is examined by two nominated medical examiners. If the recommendation is that he is not fit to practise:
3. The doctor is treated, then allowed to practise under supervision and with voluntary restrictions where necessary. He is then reassessed and if he is still not fit, then he is given further rehabilitation. If he continues to practise:
4. He is referred to the Health Committee (HC) who can suspend

him for up to 1 year or impose conditions on his practice for up to 3 years, but the HC cannot erase him. HC proceedings are heard in private but the doctor can be legally represented.

PROFESSIONAL PERFORMANCE

The Committee on Professional Performance (CPP) was established by the *Medical (Professional Performance) Act 1995* and deals with doctors whose professional performance, while poor or inadequate, does not constitute serious misconduct. It consists of a chairman who is medically qualified, four elected, one appointed and two lay members with an adviser from the relevant specialty. Its main aim is to protect the public and provide remedial action for such doctors.

Cases are usually brought to the attention of the preliminary performance screener through complaints, but may come from concerned colleagues. He must then decide whether or not formal assessment of the doctor's professional knowledge, skills and attitude towards patients and colleagues is required. If the practitioner refuses to be assessed, then he may be referred to the Assessment Referral Committee (ARC) to decide whether or not the refusal is justified. The ARC consists of three members, of which one is lay. If the ARC considers that the refusal is not justified, it can insist on the assessment by making it a condition of registration.

If assessment is recommended, then the procedure is then as follows:

1. Assessment at the place of work by three assessors (one lay and two medical from the same specialty) to identify any areas of serious deficiency
2. Remedial education and training in those areas by the appropriate Regional Postgraduate Dean or Regional Adviser in General Practice
3. Reassessment after training with the timing decided by the preliminary performance screener.

The case is then concluded or the doctor is recommended for further training and reassessment. If the doctor does not improve, then he is referred to the CPP. The practitioner can attend the hearing by the CPP and be legally represented. The CPP can suspend registration for 1 year or attach conditions for 3 years. It cannot erase, although after 2 years registration may be suspended indefinitely.

REVALIDATION

In response to public demands to make professional self-regulation more transparent and accountable, the GMC has agreed to introduce periodic revalidation, linked to registration. All doctors on the register after 2002 will have to submit evidence that they are practising within clearly defined guidelines at 5-yearly intervals. The methods of assessment are currently under debate but are likely to include a 'folder and appraisal' system.

THE NURSING AND MIDWIFERY COUNCIL (NMC)

A new regulatory body – the Nursing and Midwifery Council (NMC) – replaced the United Kingdom Central Council (UKCC) and the National Boards in April 2002. New statutory legislation (the *Nursing and Midwifery Order 2001*) was enacted and UKCC staff became NMC staff. The NMC will fulfil the same core functions as the UKCC in regard to maintaining a register of UK nurses, midwives and health visitors, providing guidance and handling professional misconduct complaints.

MAINTENANCE OF THE REGISTER

Only the NMC can grant or remove registration and it maintains the register of nurses, midwives and health visitors in a fashion similar to that of the GMC, although this register is divided into 15 parts:

1. First level nurses trained in general nursing (RGN/SRN)
2. Second level (England and Wales) (ENG/SEN)
3. First level nurses trained in nursing mental illness (RMN)
4. Second level (England and Wales) (ENM/SEN(M))
5. First level nurses trained in nursing learning disabilities (RNMH/RNMS)
6. Second level (England and Wales) (ENMH/SEN(MH))
7. All second level nurses (Scotland and Northern Ireland) (EN)

8. Nurses trained in nursing sick children (RSCN)
9. Nurses trained in nursing fever (RFN)
10. Midwives (RM)
11. Health visitors (RHV)
12. First level nurses trained in adult nursing (Project 2000) (RN – adult)
13. First level nurses trained in mental health nursing (Project 2000) (RN – mental health)
14. First level nurses trained in learning disabilities nursing (Project 2000) (RN – learning disabilities)
15. First level nurses trained in children's nursing (Project 2000) (RN – sick children).

The necessary registrable qualifications are given in parentheses.

MONITORING OF PROFESSIONAL DEVELOPMENT

Under the NMC, continuing professional development is linked to registration through PREP (post-registration education and practice). In order to maintain registration under PREP, nurses must:

- complete a notification of practice form at re-registration every 3 years or on change of area of practice to one requiring a different registrable qualification
- complete at least 35 hours of learning activity every 3 years
- maintain a personal professional profile, which is a record of career progress and professional development

- complete a return to practice programme if they have not been in practice for at least 750 hours in the previous 5 years.

PRODUCTION OF CODES, STANDARDS AND GUIDELINES FOR PRACTICE

Possibly the most important code of the NMC (UKCC 1992, see further reading) is the *Code of Professional Conduct* as it is against this that complaints of misconduct are judged. The guidelines are designed to help registrants maintain good practice (e.g. administration of medicines and record keeping).

PROFESSIONAL CONDUCT PROCEEDINGS

The *Nurses, Midwives and Health Visitors Act 1992* created the same three committees as the *Health Act 1983* and sets the NMC a statutory obligation to investigate and deal with allegations of misconduct or unfitness to practise. Complaints can come from any source but they must be in writing and they must be sufficiently serious to justify erasure from the register. As for the GMC, the police are required to notify the NMC if a registered nurse, midwife or health visitor is convicted of *any* criminal offence.

Complaints alleging misconduct are considered in private by the Preliminary Proceedings Committee (PPC), comprised of NMC Council members. The accused practitioner is informed of the allegation and invited to submit a written reply, but he is not usually asked to attend unless he is likely to be suspended.

The PPC can:

- close the case with no further action taken
- issue a caution – this is usually applied where misconduct has been proven but there are mitigating circumstances and there is no risk to the public. The caution remains on record for 5 years
- refer the case to the Panel of Screeners for consideration of a hearing before the Health Committee if the complaint demonstrates unfitness to practise by reason of ill health
- refer the case to the Professional Conduct Committee (PCC) for an oral hearing. The PPC can also apply an interim suspension if there is evidence of serious risk to either patients or the practitioner, but this is rare and usually involves criminal offences. The suspension must be reviewed every 3 months or sooner if the practitioner requests it.

PCC hearings are adversarial and are held in public. Each PCC consists of five people: three NMC Council members, a member of the consumer panel and a practitioner from the same area of practice. There is also a legal assessor to advise on points of law. The accused practitioner can be legally represented and the PCC has legal assessors available for advice. Evidence is given on oath and must

be oral, except in exceptional circumstances. The PCC must decide whether or not the facts have been proved *beyond reasonable doubt* and if they constitute misconduct. This includes: physical or verbal abuse of a patient; stealing from patients; concealing critical incidents (e.g. drug errors) and falsifying records.

The PCC must:

- conclude the case and take no further action
- postpone determination as for the GMC
- refer the case to the HC
- issue a caution or conditions on practice
- suspend the practitioner for up to 1 year
- erase him from the register either indefinitely or for a specified period.

UNFITNESS TO PRACTISE PROCEEDINGS

The NMC deals only with practitioners whose condition is serious enough to justify removing or suspending their registration to protect patients. If the practitioner voluntarily stops working, then the NMC does not need to be informed. The Panel of Screeners will only consider written allegations of unfitness to practise where the accused is identified and they have been provided with brief details of the illness. The accused must then sign a statutory declaration before the investigation can continue. The practitioner is then examined by at least two specialist medical examiners and, on the basis of their findings, the case is either dismissed or referred to either the Health Committee (HC) or back to the PPC or PCC. The accused may read the medical reports and ask for an independent report to be done if he disagrees with the findings.

The HC consists of five NMC Council members, joined by a legal assessor and a medical examiner. HC proceedings are held in private and they must decide whether or not the practitioner poses a danger to patients. If so, the HC can reach the same conclusions as the PCC, including suspension or erasure from the register. As for doctors, the commonest reasons for erasure are drug or alcohol dependence or mental illness.

RESTORATION TO THE REGISTER

The practitioner has a right to apply for restoration at any time but it is unlikely to be considered for less than a year or until after the specified period has elapsed. Such cases are heard by the PCC or the HC as appropriate and the NMC President usually chairs the hearings. If removal followed conviction for a serious criminal offence, then restoration is very unlikely. In order to be restored, the practitioner must show that he:

1. understands and accepts the reason for his removal
2. has taken appropriate action to address the problem
3. has been working in a related field for a significant time period with exemplary conduct and impeccable references.

COUNCIL FOR PROFESSIONS SUPPLEMENTARY TO MEDICINE (CPSM)

The *Professions Supplementary to Medicine Act 1960* provided a statutory and framework for the registration, regulation, training and discipline of:

- radiographers
- physiotherapists
- occupational therapists
- chiropodists
- orthoptists
- dieticians
- medical laboratory scientific officers.

Each profession has its own Board and the work of these Boards is coordinated by the CPSM. This has 23 members: an independent chairman, one member for each profession, six doctors and nine that are not members of any of the professions regulated by the Act, of which four are appointed by the Secretary of State and five by the Privy Council.

HOSPITAL DISCIPLINARY PROCEDURES

All healthcare professionals are bound by the same moral and ethical principles that apply to the general public but they also have special responsibilities. This means that any allegation of misconduct must be categorized as follows, in order to decide the most appropriate line of investigation:

- *Professional misconduct*, where the behaviour arises during the exercise of clinical skills, e.g. illegal drug prescribing or breach of confidentiality
- *Personal misconduct*, where the behaviour is unrelated to clinical skills, e.g. sexual harassment or fraud
- *Professional incompetence*, which is inadequate or poor performance of clinical skills or judgement, e.g. neglect of duties or poor record keeping.

Each Trust has its own standard form of employment contract and locally agreed internal disciplinary procedures, but the following procedures are common to most Trusts:

- For cases of personal misconduct, the procedures apply to *all* NHS employees including the provisions for the calling of witnesses, final addresses and mitigation.
- Incidents alleging professional misconduct or incompetence involve procedures unique to healthcare professionals. If the Trust does not have locally agreed procedures, then it must follow those set out in Health Circular HC(90)9 (Disciplinary procedures for Hospital and Community Medical and Dental Staff) 1990.
- Allegations can come from any source and must be thoroughly investigated prior to any disciplinary action.
- The investigating officer may be the immediate line manager (e.g. the consultant), but for clinical staff, it is often the Medical Director or even the Chief Executive.
- If the incident is serious, demonstrates a pattern of poor performance or it does not appear possible to resolve the matter locally, then the case can be referred directly to the GMC or the NMC.
- If the allegation also involves a police investigation (e.g. theft), then the disciplinary procedure can still proceed up to and including dismissal.
- If there are concerns, particularly involving the safety of patients, then the healthcare professional may be suspended during the investigation (see below).
- There must be a disciplinary hearing before any further action and the employee has a right to be informed in writing of the time, date and place, allegations, rights of representation and to bring own witnesses. This must be at least 4 days in advance and any documentary evidence and a list of witnesses must be provided not less than 2 days in advance.

- The healthcare professional can be accompanied by a friend or a union representative, but they cannot act in a legal capacity.
- The Panel usually consists of the immediate line manager or the Medical Director and a manager from Human Resources.
- The case is presented by the investigating officer with any witnesses, then the accused states his case and calls any witnesses.
- The procedure is adversarial and interrogative.
- The Panel then decides on any disciplinary action. Their decision must be confirmed in writing within 7 days, stating the rights of appeal. The following types of action are available:
  — Nothing proven, in which case, no action is taken
  — Resolution on an informal basis – this usually involves a meeting between the parties concerned with a reassessment of the situation after 3–6 months
  — Counselling
  — *Oral warning* – this is for first-time minor offences
  — *Written warning* – this is for more serious offences or a second minor offence within 3 months (e.g. constant lateness) and can stay on the personal file for up to 1 year
  — *Final written warning* – this is

Note

Warnings on records are not transferable between Trusts, only within, but beware of the 'old-boy' network!

for more than one serious offence in a year and stays on the file for up to 18 months.

SERIOUS OFFENCES

- If the Panel decides that the allegation is serious, for example misuse of controlled drugs or violent behaviour, then the healthcare professional must be informed (verbally and in writing) by the Chairman of Trust that a formal Inquiry Panel is to be set up. The healthcare professional must also be sent copies of all relevant correspondence and a list of witnesses for the 'prosecution' with a note of the main points on which they can give evidence. This must be received at least 21 days in advance of his appearance before the Panel.
- The Inquiry Panel consists of a legally qualified chairman nominated by the Lord Chancellor, plus two others. If the allegation is of professional misconduct, then they are a doctor (or nurse) and a lay person; if it is alleged incompetence, then they are both doctors (or nurses) with at least one coming from the same specialty. Note that the healthcare professional has no influence on this and these panel members may not necessarily favour the same policies and practices or they may even be known antagonists. The lay person is generally a non-executive from the Trust Board with legal experience. Once appointed, the Panel should meet within 3 months.

- The proceedings are adversarial, interrogative and held in private. Evidence is given on oath and the healthcare professional is entitled to legal representation.
- The standard of proof required is the civil standard, i.e. the *balance of probabilities,* so making it flexible, but the standard goes higher with the increasing seniority of the practitioner. The burden of proof is on the Trusty.
- The hearing should be concluded within 1 week and the Panel then must produce a report within 4 weeks, stating the findings of fact and the details of the practitioners (if any) who are at fault.
- Note that the Panel has no disciplinary powers.
- The practitioner is sent a copy of the report and he is given an opportunity to make further representations to the Trust within 4 weeks. He can request amendments that are either implemented or, if the Panel does not agree, appended to the report. He can also provide additional evidence and request a further hearing.
- The whole report is then sent to the Trust Board within 4 weeks and they decide what action, if any, to take. This includes:
  — *Dismissal with notice* – this is for a very serious offence, e.g. drug abuse *but where the welfare of patients has not been put in jeopardy;* the length of notice given depends on the contract
  — *Action short of dismissal* – for example transfer to other work or to a different location that may result in lower pay or lesser conditions of service. This may include up to 4 weeks of unpaid leave
  — *Summary dismissal* – this is immediate dismissal without notice, for example gross misconduct such as theft or assault or where the welfare of the patients has been put in jeopardy. This includes dereliction of duty and drug or alcohol abuse. Junior grades of staff can be summarily dismissed by their seniors, usually in the presence of a senior Human Resources officer.

APPEALS

- Healthcare professionals can appeal against any action but this must be sent to the Director of Human Resources within 21 days.
- The appeal is heard by a committee of three Trust Board members, of which at least one must have specialist knowledge.
- If a doctor or dentist was appointed before the Trust was formed, he can appeal to the Secretary of State under Section 190 of HC(90)9 but the notice of appeal must be lodged *before* the date that the dismissal takes effect.
- The Secretary of State must ask the Trust for their written views within 2 months and set up a professional committee to advise him. The committee can hold a hearing or make their decision on the basis of written evidence alone.
- The committee then reports to the Secretary of State, advising termination or continuance of

employment or some other solution acceptable to both the Trust and the practitioner, e.g. re-employment in another post.

- The Secretary of State must make his decision within 3 months.

SUSPENSION FROM DUTY

Suspension is the most immediate, humiliating and professionally damaging consequence of any allegation made against a healthcare professional although it should be seen as a 'neutral act' to protect the interests of patients, other staff or the practitioner and/or to assist the investigative process. Where suspension is the only solution, then the framework set out Health Service Guidelines HSG(94)49 must be followed to avoid its misuse and to minimize its length.

All suspensions should be done in private with a witness present and immediately confirmed in writing. Allegations leading to suspension should be substantiated within 10 days and the suspension should be reviewed every 2 weeks, with the practitioner being informed of the outcome. The investigation should be completed within 3 months or reasons given to the Trust Board. Suspension applies to all grades of healthcare professional and the only recourse is an industrial tribunal – there is no legal remedy, as it is not regarded in law as very damaging, since the healthcare professional is on full pay throughout. Note that doctors suspended by the NHS can continue to practise in the private sector until their registration is affected.

PREMATURE RETIREMENT

Under Health Service Guidelines HSG(95)25, NHS Trusts can retire a doctor prematurely on the grounds of the 'efficiency of the service'. This procedure applies to doctors whose performance has shown a consistent decline to an unacceptable level and which is considered unlikely to improve despite appropriate remedial action. It may be preceded by a period of 'gardening leave', where the doctor is given leave on full pay for a period not usually exceeding 6 months. It is usually used for sick doctors (e.g. alcoholic or dementing) and it theoretically allows time for the doctor to 'recover from illness' but he is rarely reinstated.

INDUSTRIAL TRIBUNALS

- These provide a limited remedy for racial and sexual discrimination and unfair dismissal, including 'constructive dismissal'. This is behaviour of an employer such that an employee is entitled to terminate his employment and consider himself dismissed, e.g. being instructed to work in a different hospital from that to which he is contracted.
- The healthcare professional must have been employed by the Trust for more than 2 years and must make his application within 3 months of the date of dismissal.
- The Trust must show that the dismissal was fair (i.e. the burden of proof is on the Trust) and for this to be true, the dismissal must be based on:

— capability or qualification
— misconduct
— restriction imposed by statute, e.g. loss of registration
— redundancy
— some other substantial reason.

- The fundamental inadequacy of an industrial tribunal is that if the healthcare professional is found to have been unfairly dismissed, he may not *necessarily* get his job back as the tribunal cannot enforce the order for reinstatement. It can only 'fine' the employer by making them pay an additional award to the employee on top of the normal compensation, which is a basic award of years of service (up to a maximum of 20) multiplied by their weekly wage.

THE 'THREE WISE MEN' PROCEDURE

- This was designed to help prevent harm to patients resulting from physical or mental disability of medical or dental staff, including locums, as set out in Health Circular HC(82)13.
- It advises each Trust to set up a special professional panel of senior medical and dental staff from which, on a case-by-case basis, a subcommittee of three members can be appointed 'to take action on any report of incapacity due to physical or mental disability including addiction'.
- The panel is usually chaired by the Chairman of the Hospital Medical Staff Committee.
- The panel receives an allegation of disability and makes confidential inquiries to verify the accuracy of the report.
- If it has substance, the practitioner is given the opportunity to be interviewed with either a colleague or a representative from his defence organization present.
- The panel then reports to the Chairman of the Trust who decides on further action, which can include referral to the GMC Health Committee.
- There are similar arrangements for general practitioners, operated by the local medical committee, but they are informal and have never been properly evaluated.

DISCIPLINARY PROCEDURES IN GENERAL PRACTICE

- General practitioners are independent contractors, so they cannot be suspended by health authorities, even in serious circumstances.
- Allegations of poor performance are usually dealt with by the local medical committee but they may not be effective in resolving serious problems and the procedures have no statutory basis.

- Note that there is no facility for suspending or otherwise dealing with the poor performance of doctors who work within general practice but are not principals, e.g. clinical assistants and locums. These doctors can only be dismissed under employment law procedures and dismissal from one practice or deputizing service often leaves the doctor free to seek employment elsewhere.
- General practitioners can only be removed from NHS practice by either the GMC or via the NHS Tribunal.

THE NHS TRIBUNAL

- This is a public body set up under section 46 of the *NHS Act 1977* and is empowered by the *Tribunals and Inquiries Act 1992*.
- The complainant must be an administrative body, e.g. a Trust or the GMC, and it must produce a concise statement of the facts and reasons why the doctor or dentist should not continue to practise.

- Complaints are received directly by the legally qualified chairman and if he considers that a complaint has substance, he sets up a tribunal.
- The process is inquisitorial so only oral evidence is considered and this is given on oath. The burden of proof is the criminal standard and the doctor or dentist is entitled to legal representation.
- The tribunal can order an interim suspension or can disqualify the practitioner but it is often a very lengthy process.
- Note that disqualification means that the practitioner can no longer work as a principal but, theoretically, he can still work in an NHS hospital or in the private sector, unlike being taken off the GMC register.
- Appearance before a tribunal is very rare and usually occurs only after the practitioner has committed a series of breaches of his contract. However, it is also extremely rare to be reinstated as this involves an appeal process to court for a judicial review to prove that the tribunal was illegal.

NATIONAL CLINICAL ASSESSMENT AGENCY (NCAA)

This is a new special health authority established in April 2001 in order to provide a fast response when an NHS employer or, for general practitioners, a health authority, raises concerns about a doctor's performance that cannot be resolved locally. The aim is to remove the need for long suspensions and to provide a central point of advice. The health authority or the employer will retain responsibility for any action taken but, following assessment, the NCAA can make the following recommendations:

- No action required
- Practise while being monitored against set criteria
- A period of retraining followed by reassessment
- Reskilling in a different field followed by reassessment

- Referral to the GMC
- Referral for medical treatment
- Referral back to the employer or health authority with a report that the problem is serious and intractable.

DEALING WITH A COLLEAGUE WHO IS UNDERPERFORMING

- Wherever possible, discuss your concerns with your colleague directly and preferably face-to-face, although a letter or telephone call may be easier.
- If this is not feasible, ask another healthcare professional who is known to be a close friend of the person concerned to speak to him as this may make him less defensive and more able to seek help.
- If the problem appears to be related to his health, and the safety of patients may be at risk, try to contact his general practitioner.
- If the problem is not health related, you can voice your concerns to his immediate senior, the local medical committee (for general practitioners), the Clinical or Medical Director (for consultants), the Director of Nursing or the Chief Executive of the Trust.
- If local resolution is either inappropriate or unsatisfactory, the problem is obviously serious or the healthcare professional has committed a criminal offence, then you should contact the NMC

or the GMC as appropriate.
- In all cases, you must inform the person concerned of your actions but limit any information given to those who must know in order to investigate the matter further or you may be vulnerable to an action for slander or libel.
- Make sure that your facts are accurate and verifiable but note that any clinical records used should not identify the patient unless it is unavoidable.
- Try to be objective and make any potential conflict of interest known, e.g. a pre-existing disagreement with the person concerned.
- Note that both the GMC and the NMC have stated that healthcare professionals have an 'ethical responsibility to act where they believe a colleague's conduct, performance or health is a threat to patients and if they ignore this responsibility, they put themselves at risk of action by their disciplinary body.
- Under the *Public Interest Disclosure Act 1998,* you cannot be victimized, subjected to a detriment, dismissed or made

redundant after making a 'protected disclosure', i.e. only to the relevant bodies. The disclosure must concern matters of public interest, such as criminal offences or health and safety concerns, and be made in good faith, so it cannot be anonymous. If the concerns are not acted upon or if you believe that you are being victimized, then you can legitimately take your concerns externally, for example to the police, media or the Department of Health. However, this must be considered 'reasonable' by any subsequent tribunal and must not breach patient confidentiality. If you are sacked, then you can apply for an interim order to keep your job before appearing before a tribunal. If you are then found to have been unfairly dismissed, then you will be eligible for unlimited compensation.

Reference

1. General Medical Council. Protecting patients: a summary consultative document. London: GMC, 2001

Further reading

Department of Health. Disciplinary procedures for hospital and community medical and dental staff (HC(90)9). London: DoH, 1990

General Medical Council. Good medical practice. London: GMC, 1998

General Medical Council. Maintaining good medical practice. London: GMC, 1998

United Kingdom Central Council. Code of professional conduct. London: UKCC, 1992

United Kingdom Central Council. Scope of professional practice. London: UKCC, 1992

Useful websites

General Medical Council: www.gmc-uk.org
Nursing and Midwifery Council: www.nmc.org.uk

CHAPTER 11

DEATH AND THE HEALTHCARE PROFESSIONAL

INTRODUCTION

As will be discussed in Chapter 12, there is no statutory definition of death in the United Kingdom and the diagnosis of death remains a matter of clinical judgement. When a person is thought to have died, a doctor will be called to 'certify the body'. However, as the doctor may issue a death certificate only under very limited circumstances, it is more accurate to describe the process as 'confirming death'. If that death has occurred outside the hospital, the doctor may also be asked for an estimation of the time of death and whether or not he feels that there are any suspicious circumstances (e.g. a potential murder or suicide). This often causes some concern so this chapter will cover the procedures involved. It will then discuss the role, courts and verdicts of the Coroner and the Procurator Fiscal.

CONFIRMATION OF DEATH

In the past, doctors were always called to confirm death but they have *no legal obligation* to:

1. confirm death
2. view the dead body
3. report the fact of a death – although a doctor must report the *cause* of death if he attended the deceased during the final illness.

This means that there have been significant changes in who is allowed to confirm death. The NMC now advise that a registered nurse can confirm death in situations where the death is *expected* and where there is an explicit local policy or protocol to allow such an action (e.g. nursing homes). The nurse must have received appropriate training prior to taking on this additional role. In some areas, paramedics have also been given the power to confirm death.

DEATHS OUT OF HOSPITAL

As a healthcare professional, you have no statutory or contractual requirement to attend a dead body, but if you are a general practitioner you do have a moral obligation to attend as soon as practicable if it is that of one of the patients on your list. If the person is not registered with you, then most local medical committees advise that you should ask that the Forensic Medical Examiner be called instead.

ON ARRIVAL

- If the death is expected, confirm death (see below) and inform those in attendance that they can contact the undertaker. If you are able to sign the Medical Certificate of Cause of Death (see below), then do so.
- If the death is unexpected but there are no suspicious circumstances, confirm death (see below) and inform the Coroner, either through the Coroner's Officer or the police. Do not sign a certificate until agreed by the Coroner. Tell those in attendance that the Coroner's Officer will either arrange for the body to be removed or allow them to call the undertaker.
- If the death is unexpected and there appear to be suspicious circumstances, call the police. If they are already present, then talk to the officer in charge as you must not disturb or contaminate any potential evidence during your examination. This in turn may be much more limited and only done once the scene has been photographed. You will also be shown the route to follow when approaching and leaving the body.

Remember! The police can investigate any scene that they consider suspicious but if *you* state that you believe that the cause of death was not natural, then they *must* investigate the scene further.

TAKE A HISTORY

This may come from the police and/or the relatives. Try to ascertain:

- *when and where the person was last seen or heard and by whom.* This will give you clues when trying to estimate how long the person has been dead. It may also be useful in deciding whether or not there are suspicious circumstances, for example the relative who claims to have seen the person the day before when life has obviously been extinct for much longer
- *how and where the body was discovered and by whom.* The body should not have been moved but this is not always the case, particularly if attempts have been made at resuscitation by the relatives or ambulance personnel
- *any relevant past medical or surgical history.* This may help in establishing the cause of death although this is *not* your role, other than giving an opinion as to whether it was natural or not.

NOTE THE SURROUNDINGS

Detailed crime scene investigation is the role of the police but it is useful to note the following:

- signs of forced entry, other than those caused by the police who have a power of entry if they consider that lives may be at risk
- medication, including empty bottles
- drug paraphernalia, e.g. 'crack' pipes, syringes

- signs of alcohol abuse, e.g. empty cans and bottles
- signs of neglect
- the temperature of the room (see below)
- the dates of any newspapers or letters.

EXAMINE THE BODY

As stated, your examination may be limited to observation only and if so, you should note:

- any obvious injuries, particularly potentially lethal wounds, defence injuries or signs of previous self-harm. Describe them accurately in your notes (see Ch. 3)
- any signs of struggle
- the site and position of the body
- the condition and position of any clothing
- any blood or vomit around the mouth and nose
- signs of post mortem hypostasis (see below)
- potential instruments of murder or suicide, e.g. a ligature around the neck
- any stigmata of chronic disease, e.g. spider naevi in liver disease
- any obvious scars, particularly surgical ones.

If you are allowed to touch the body, then also check:

- the temperature of the body (see below)
- any movement in the small and large joints (see below)
- for any hidden injuries, marks or scars, provided you can turn the body over.

CONFIRM DEATH

Death in situations other than those described in Chapter 12 is usually confirmed by noting the absence of the carotid pulse, breath and heart sounds. If the person has only recently died, then you must listen to the chest for several minutes as there are many conditions that may mimic death (e.g. hypothermia, coma and drug overdoses). It is distressing to note that in the home situation, the person has often been dead for weeks to months and there is rarely any doubt regarding the fact that the person is dead. However, mistakes have been made and you must be absolutely certain that life is extinct before sending the body to the mortuary.

STATE THE TIME OF DEATH

The legal date and time of death is that which you state on completion of your examination of the body, even if you believe that the person actually died months earlier.

TALK TO THE RELATIVES

If there are relatives present, it is important to talk to them. Be sympathetic and, if there are no suspicious circumstances, then reassure them that there was nothing else that could have been done to save their relative. It is vital to try to help them with the guilt that they inevitably feel and even if you think that earlier medical intervention might have changed the outcome, there is *nothing* to be gained from expressing this belief. If possible, tell them that you think that their relative did not suffer but do not try to guess at the cause of death unless you are in a position to issue a certificate (see below). Warn them if you think that a post mortem will be necessary but reassure them that it should not interfere with their funeral arrangements unless there is any suspicion that the cause of death was not natural. Ask them if they have any further questions before leaving but if you do not know the answer, admit it.

DEATHS IN HOSPITAL

Confirming death in hospital is much simpler as there are rarely suspicious circumstances, although this may occur, such as the psychiatric patient who successfully commits suicide. You may be asked to confirm death in the back of the ambulance so that the patient can be taken directly to the mortuary but this should never be done if there are relatives present unless there is no hope of resuscitation (e.g. a person decapitated in a road accident). Even when confirming death in a ward patient, you should still take a history as above and also refer to the hospital notes. You must examine the body thoroughly prior to confirming death, as a death in hospital does not necessarily equate to a death from natural causes.

ESTIMATION OF TIME OF DEATH

This is a subject of much debate and while the following may give clues towards the likely time of death, none is 100% accurate and you should not be too dogmatic in your estimate. There are many good books on the subject (see Further reading) so the following provides an outline only.

RIGOR MORTIS

After death, the muscle glycogen stores start to deplete and adenosine triphosphate (ATP) can no longer be resynthesized from adenosine diphosphate (ADP). This results in a sustained contraction in all the muscles with subsequent stiffness, known as rigor mortis. The effects are most pronounced in the small muscles initially, so the jaw, finger and toe joints are affected first. As the process continues, the larger joints such as the hips, knees and elbows become affected. As time progresses, the muscles then start to deteriorate, the contracture decreases and the body becomes flaccid again. The onset of rigor mortis is very variable and is affected by factors such as the ambient temperature – it occurs earlier with higher temperatures – and the level of initial glycogen stores, so it starts earlier if the person was very active prior to death (e.g. struggling or fitting). Generally, the duration of rigor mortis follows the pattern shown in Table 11.1 but its use in determining the time of death is limited by the variation.

Cadaveric spasm is an extreme variant that occurs immediately after death. The mechanism is not understood but it is more common in people who have suffered a severe 'fight or flight' reaction just prior to death (e.g. soldiers). Fire victims may be found in a 'pugilistic attitude', where their stance suggests that they are about to punch someone. This is caused by heat contractures within the flexor muscles.

POST MORTEM HYPOSTASIS

This is also known as lividity and occurs as a result of gravitational pooling of blood. It looks similar to bruising and is seen in dependent areas of the body although pressure points are paler due to sparing. It also has a very variable onset but usually starts about an hour after death and becomes complete after 6–12 hours. It then becomes 'fixed' and remains unchanged until putrefaction occurs. The variability in onset means that it cannot be accurately used to assess time of death but if it is seen in non-dependent areas, it suggests that the body was moved after death. It may be very faint if the death was preceded by massive haemorrhage. The normal colour is blue/red but different colours may give an idea of the cause of death (Table 11.2).

TEMPERATURE

Traditional teaching states that the body temperature declines at a rate of 0.9°C per hour after death but this is inaccurate as body cooling occurs in a sigmoid fashion, not linear, and varies with many different factors, such as:

- clothing
- ambient temperature, humidity and air movement

TABLE 11.1	Pattern of rigor mortis
Time of death	Pattern
< 3 hours	Body is warm and flaccid
3–6 hours	The small muscles contract and the jaw, toe and finger joints stiffen
6–12 hours	The larger muscles contract and the hip, knee and elbow joints stiffen
12–18 hours	Rigor mortis is complete
18–36 hours	The muscles start to deteriorate and the small, then large joints become mobile
> 36 hours	Body is cold and flaccid

TABLE 11.2 Relevance of colour of lividity		
Colour	Caused by	Likely cause of death
Cherry red	Carboxyhaemoglobin	Carbon monoxide poisoning
Pink	Undissociated oxyhaemoglobin	Hypothermia
Dark red	Oxygenated blood	Cyanide poisoning
Grey-brown	Methaemoglobinaemia	Ethylene glycol poisoning (antifreeze)

- body temperature immediately before death, e.g. fever
- body fat or oedema, which acts as an insulator
- immersion.

A rectal thermometer is more likely to give an accurate reading than a surface one but this may interfere with the forensic evidence so it should not be done at the scene. Any comments regarding the temperature of the body are best limited to whether the body feels cold or warm to the touch.

DECOMPOSITION

Putrefaction is the process by which the body disintegrates tissue. It also has a very variable time of onset and depends on many factors, such as:

- ambient temperature – the hotter the surroundings, the quicker the onset
- body fat or oedema, which hastens putrefaction
- burial or immersion in water, which delays the changes.

Putrefaction starts as a greenish discolouration of the right iliac fossa over the caecum on the third day. This spreads and reaches the face by about 7 days, when the skin starts to blister and erode. Gas formation starts in the softer tissues around the neck, abdomen and genitals, and involves the whole body by the end of the second week. In warm, humid surroundings, the body fat may be converted to a waxy substance called 'adipocere', which may persist for years. If the body is in warm, dry surroundings, it can mummify and become brown and leathery.

OTHER METHODS

Other methods of determining the time of death include:

- *Biochemical* – changes in the blood, urine and cerebrospinal fluid
- *Eye changes* – segmentation in the retinal blood vessels, corneal opacity and dark marks on the sclera ('taches noires sclerotiques')
- *Entomology* – the presence or absence of different types of maggots and other parasites
- *Botany* – growth of different types of plants through interred or concealed bodies.

DEATH CERTIFICATION IN ENGLAND AND WALES

Certification of death must be done accurately and promptly as it provides legal evidence of the fact and cause of death. This allows the death to be registered so that the family can make arrangement to dispose of the body and the data can be used for mortality statistics. About 75% of deaths in the United Kingdom are certified by a doctor and the remainder by a Coroner/Procurator Fiscal. There are three types of certificate:

- *Stillbirth Certificate* (after 24 weeks' gestation) – this is completed by the doctor or midwife present at the birth
- *Neonatal Death Certificate* (any death up to 28 days of age)
- *Medical Certificate of Cause of Death* – also known as the 'death certificate' (all other deaths; see Fig. 11.1)

Under Section 22 of the *Births and Deaths Registration Act 1953,* a doctor who has attended the deceased during his last illness must sign the death certificate, stating the cause of death to the 'best of his knowledge and belief' *unless* the death is one that should be reported to the Coroner. As shown in Figure 11.1, the form is divided into three parts:

- The left side is a counterfoil to be retained by the doctor for his records
- The right side is a 'Notice to Informant', which confirms that the certificate has been issued to the relatives or other authorized persons. Note that this part is absent on the forms used in Northern Ireland and Scotland
- The centre part is the actual certificate. This must be taken to the Registrar within 5 days.

COMPLETING A MEDICAL CERTIFICATE OF CAUSE

If you are asked to complete such a certificate, you should note the following:

- You must be a registered medical practitioner (full or provisional) and you must have attended the deceased during his last illness. You must also have seen the deceased either after or within 14 days of the death. If you have seen him in the preceding 14 days, then there is no *legal* requirement for you to see the body after death before you complete the certificate but it is good practice so to do.
- The most important part of the certificate is the actual cause of death, which is divided into Parts I and II. Part I should indicate the disease or condition directly leading to the death, and II, any contributing diseases not directly related to the condition causing the death, e.g. Part I might be ischaemic heart disease and Part II, diabetes or smoking.

- Do not record the mode of death and never give it as the cause of death, e.g. heart failure or uraemia.
- Never use abbreviations as this can lead to ambiguity, e.g. M.S. may mean mitral stenosis, multiple sclerosis or Marfan's syndrome.
- You can now give 'old age' as a cause of death but only if you cannot give a more specific cause and the deceased was over 70.
- Do not withhold sensitive information in deference to the relatives, e.g. that the deceased had AIDS (see Ch. 6).
- Note that death from AIDS or in an HIV-positive person does not need to be referred to the Coroner unless there are other grounds.
- Refer to the notes and directions contained in the book of certificates as these are a useful source of help and advice. The books are held in either the general practitioner surgery or the Bereavement Office at the hospital.
- If you are in hospital, you must give the name of the consultant in charge of the patient. This is because the Registrar may require further information in the future and junior staff change frequently.
- If you issue a certificate in a case that you wish to report to the Coroner, initial Box A on the back of the certificate. This will alert the Registrar but you will also need to talk to the Coroner directly.
- If you wish to wait for the results of tests prior to categorizing the death, initial Box B on the back of the form. There is also a space on

the front of the form to indicate that the results of a post mortem may be available later.
- If in doubt, discuss the case with the Coroner's Officer.

There is no *statutory* duty for a doctor to report *any* death to the Coroner – this duty lies with the Registrar. However, it is good practice to report all deaths occurring within 24 hours of admission to hospital and also those that the Registrar must report, as shown in the box below.

Deaths that must be reported to the Coroner

- The cause of death is unknown even if the doctor was in regular attendance
- The deceased was not attended by a doctor during his last illness
- The deceased was not seen by the attending doctor either after death or within the 14 days before death
- The death was violent, suspicious or unnatural
- All forms of injury, ill treatment, starvation and poisoning, whether the death occurred as a direct or indirect result, e.g. following surgery or infection
- Accidental deaths
- Deaths that may have been due to neglect – either by self or others
- Deaths that may have been caused by industrial disease or related to employment
- Deaths following an abortion
- Suicides
- Deaths that occurred during an operation or before recovery from the anaesthetic
- Deaths in custody

MED A
14 000000

COUNTERFOIL

For use of Medical Practitioner, who should complete in all cases

Name of deceased

Date of death

Place of death

Last seen alive by me

Post-mortem?/* 1 2 3 4

Coroner

Whether seen after death* a b c

Cause of death:

I

(a)

(b)

(c)

II

Employment? [ ] Please tick where applicable

B Further information offered?

Signature

Date

* *Ring appropriate digit(s) and letter*

MED A
14 000000

Registrar to enter
No. of Death Entry

BIRTHS AND DEATHS REGISTRATION ACT 1953

(Form prescribed by the Registration of Births, Deaths and Marriages (Amendment) Regulations 1968)

MEDICAL CERTIFICATE OF CAUSE OF DEATH

For use only by a registered Medical Practitioner WHO HAS BEEN IN ATTENDANCE during the deceased's last illness, and to be delivered by him forthwith to the Registrar of Births and Deaths

Name of deceased

Date of death as stated to me .... day of .... 19...... Age as stated to me ......

Place of death .... day of .... 19......

Last seen alive by me ....

1 The certified cause of death takes account of information obtained from post-mortem
2 Information from post-mortem may be available later.
3 Post-mortem not being held.
4 I have reported this death to the Coroner for further action (see overleaf).

Please ring appropriate digit(s) and letter

a Seen after death by me
b Seen after death by another medical practitioner but not by me
c Not seen after death by a medical practitioner

CAUSE OF DEATH

The condition thought to be the Underlying Cause of Death should appear in the lowest completed line of Part I

I (a) Disease or condition directly leading to death **......
(b) Other disease or condition, if any, leading to (a)......
(c) Other disease or condition, if any, leading to (b)......

II Other significant conditions CONTRIBUTING TO THE DEATH but not related to the disease or condition causing it ......

These particulars not to be entered in death register

Approximate interval between onset and death

The death might have been due to or contributed to by the employment followed at some time by the deceased. [ ] Please tick where applicable

**This does not mean the mode of dying, such as heart failure, asphyxia, asthenia, etc. It means the disease, injury, or complication which caused death.

I hereby certify that I was in medical attendance during the above named deceased's last illness, and that the particulars and cause of death above written are true to the best of my knowledge and belief

Signature ......
Qualifications as registered by General Medical Council
Residence ......
Date ......

For death in hospital: Please give the name of the consultant responsible for the above-named as a patient

---

MED A
14 000000

(Form prescribed by the Registration of Births, Deaths and Marriages Regulations 1968)

NOTICE TO INFORMANT

I hereby give notice that I have this day signed a medical certificate of cause of death of

Signature ......
Date ......

This notice is to be delivered by the informant to the registrar of births and deaths for the sub-district in which the death occurred

The certifying medical practitioner must give this notice to the person who is qualified and liable to act as informant for the registration of death (see list overleaf).

Failure to deliver this notice to the registrar renders the informant liable to prosecution. The death cannot be registered until the medical certificate has reached the registrar.

DUTIES OF INFORMANT

When the death is registered the informant must be prepared to give to the registrar the following particulars relating to the deceased:

1. The date and place of death
2. The full name and surname (and the maiden surname if the deceased was a woman who had married).
3. The date and place of birth.
4. The occupation (and if the deceased was a married woman or a widow the name and occupation of her husband).
5. The usual address.
6. Whether the deceased was in receipt of a pension or allowance from public funds.
7. If the deceased was married, the date of birth of the surviving widow or widower.

THE DECEASED'S MEDICAL CARD SHOULD BE DELIVERED TO THE REGISTRAR

Fig. 11.1 Medical Certificate of Cause of Death. (i) front of form

Complete where applicable

PERSONS QUALIFIED AND LIABLE TO ACT AS INFORMANTS

The following persons are designated by the Births and Deaths Registration Act 1953 as qualified to give information concerning a death:–

DEATHS IN HOUSES AND PUBLIC INSTITUTIONS

(1) A relative of the deceased, present at the death.

(2) A relative of the deceased, in attendance during the last illness.

(3) A relative of the deceased, residing or being in the sub-district where the death occurred.

(4) A person present at the death.

(5) The occupier* if he knew of the happening of the death.

(6) Any inmate if he knew of the happening of the death.

(7) The person causing the disposal of the body.

DEATHS IN HOUSES OR DEAD BODIES FOUND

(1) Any relative of the deceased having knowledge of any of the particulars required to be registered.

(2) Any person present at the death.

(3) Any person who found the body.

(4) Any person in charge of the body.

(5) The person causing the disposal of the body.

* 'Occupier' in relation to a public institution includes the governor, keeper, master, matron, superintendent, or other chief resident officer.

A

I have reported this death to the Coroner for further action.

Initials of certifying medical practitioner.

The Coroner needs to consider all cases where:
  The death might have been due to or contributed to by a violent or unnatural cause (including an accident);
or the cause of death cannot be identified:
or the death might have been due to or contributed to by drugs, medicine, abortion or poison:

B

I may be in a position later to give, on application by the Registrar General, additional information as to the cause of death for the purpose or more precise statistical classification.

Initials of certifying medical practitioner.

  or there is reason to believe that the death occurred during an operation or under or prior to complete recovery from an operation or an anaesthetic:
  or the death might have been due to or contributed to by the employment followed at some time by the deceased.

LIST OF SOME OF THE CATEGORIES OF DEATH WHICH MAY BE OF INDUSTRIAL ORIGIN

MALIGNANT DISEASES

		Causes include:
(a)	Skin	–radiation and sunlight –pitch tar –mineral oils
(b)	Nasal	–wood or leather work –nickel
(c)	Lungs	–asbestos –nickel –radiation
(d)	Pleura	–asbestos
(e)	Urinary Tract	–benzidine –dyestuff –chemicals in rubber –PVC manufacture
(f)	Liver	–radiation
(g)	Bone	–radiation –benzene
(h)	Lymphatics and haematopoietic	

POISONING

(a)	Metals	e.g. arsenics, cadmium, lear,
(b)	Chemicals	e.g. chlorine, benzene
(c)	Solvents	e.g. trichlorethylene

INFECTIOUS DISEASES

		Causes include:
(a)	Anthrax	imported bone, bonemeal, hide or fur
(b)	Brucellosis	farming or veterinary contact at work
(c)	Tuberculosis	farming, sewer or under- ground workers
(d)	Leptospirosis	farming or gardening
(e)	Tetanus	animal handling
(f)	Rabies	contact at work
(g)	Viral hepatitis	

BRONCHIAL ASTHMA AND PNEUMONITIS

(a)	Occupational asthma	sensitising agent at work
(b)	Allergic Alveolitis	farming

PNEUMOCONIOSIS

	mining and quarrying
	potteries
	asbestos

NOTE:—The Practitioner, on signing the certificate, should complete, sign and date the Notice to the Informant, which should be detached and handed to the Informant. The Practitioner should then, without delay, deliver the certificate itself to the Registrar of Births and Deaths for the sub-district in which the death occurred. Envelopes for enclosing the certificates are supplied by the Registrar.

Fig. 11.1 Medical Certificate of Cause of Death. (ii) back of form.

This reduces delay in registration and allows you to explain the reasons for the referral to the relatives. You should still complete the certificate unless the Coroner advises against this but be sure to initial Box A. If the deceased died from natural causes, the following may occur:

- There are no reasons to report the death to the Coroner so the doctor completes the certificate unless a post mortem is requested for clinical interest. This is done to establish the extent of the disease, not the cause of death, although a study in 2001 showed that in over 60% of cases where a post mortem was carried out for this purpose, the predicted cause of death was wrong.[1]

- The death is reported but a natural cause can be established without a post mortem and the Coroner issues a Form 100A to the Registrar. This informs him that death was due to natural causes and he advises the doctor to complete the certificate.

- A post mortem examination is deemed necessary but reveals a natural cause of death. The Coroner issues a Form 100B to the Registrar, informing him of the cause of death and that no further action is required.

Once the Registrar receives either the certificate or Form 100B, he registers the death and issues a disposal certificate. If the deceased died of unnatural causes, then an inquest must be held.

THE CORONER SYSTEM

Coroners date from 1194, but the office has evolved from a predominantly fiscal role in protecting the royal revenues to that of an independent judicial officer responsible for the investigation of all unnatural deaths occurring within his district. There are 146 Coroner's districts in England and Wales, based mostly on administrative counties, and the caseloads vary from 100–5000 reported deaths per year. Coroners can be medically (5 or more years) or legally qualified (often both). They are appointed by the local authority but can only be removed by the Lord Chancellor. The jurisdiction of the Coroner relates to the presence of the body in his district, irrespective of where the person actually died so it includes people who have died abroad but have been returned home. Under Section 8 of the *Coroners Act 1988*, the Coroner must conduct an inquest if there is reasonable cause to suspect that the death:

- was violent or unnatural
- was caused by industrial disease
- remains of unknown cause despite a post mortem
- occurred in custody.

The Coroner usually sits alone but a jury of 7–11 members joins him for:

- deaths in custody or as a result of injury caused by a police officer in the execution of his duty
- industrial deaths, including accidents, poisoning and diseases, e.g. asbestosis
- deaths that occurred in circumstances that, were they to be continued or repeated, would prove prejudicial to public safety, e.g. train crashes.

Inquests are often opened initially shortly after the death to hear evidence of the identity of the deceased and the medical cause of death, then adjourned to allow the Coroner's enquiries to be completed. Where someone has been charged with causing the death, the inquest will be adjourned until after the trial but the death will be registered. The Coroner may give permission for the body to be cremated or buried in the interim if this would not result in loss of valuable evidence.

APPEARING AT AN INQUEST

The conduct of an inquest is governed by the *Coroners Rules 1984* and it is inquisitorial in nature, unlike the adversarial approach of the remainder of the British legal systems (see Ch. 1). The Coroner decides which witnesses should be called and, whilst there is no obligation upon any witness to provide a statement in advance, it is advisable to do so if asked. Anyone can offer to give evidence or inform the Coroner that they believe that a particular witness should be called. As for any other court, the Coroner

can compel a witness to attend upon penalty of a fine or even imprisonment.

The degree of formality varies but it can be very intimidating, particularly if the family of the deceased is present, and you must dress smartly. As for the other courts, you will be expected to have brought any relevant notes, investigations and X-rays. Evidence is given under oath and you should follow the advice given in Chapter 2. You will initially be examined by the Coroner and this is usually quite neutral, merely seeking to establish the facts of the case. Hearsay evidence is allowed and you may be asked to comment on the medical notes made by others. Although many Coroners are also medically qualified, use layman's terms wherever possible so that the family can understand. You may then be questioned by anyone with a 'proper interest' as defined in the *Coroners Rules 1984* – either in person or through a legal representative.

Persons with a 'proper interest'

- Parent/spouse/child or anyone acting for the deceased
- Beneficiaries and issuers of the deceased's life insurance policy
- Anyone whose actions the Coroner believes may have contributed to the death, accidentally or otherwise.
- The Chief Police Officer (only through a lawyer)
- Governmental officials appointed to attend the inquest
- Anyone else that the Coroner decides has a 'proper interest'.

Questions must be sensible and the Coroner can insist that you answer all relevant questions unless it would result in self-incrimination of a criminal act. This questioning can be very difficult, particularly if there is a suggestion of negligence by yourself or your colleagues and you must try to remain calm and composed. Remember that the role of the inquest is solely to establish the identity of the deceased and how, when and where he died. It must not infer either criminal or civil liability on any named person although both types of proceeding may follow an inquest. You are also entitled to have legal representation and if you are concerned that your conduct may be called into question, then it is wise to have a legal adviser present. Note that legal aid is not available for inquests.

The standard of proof is the civil standard of 'balance of probabilities' *except* for the verdicts of suicide or unlawful killing, where it must be proved to the criminal standard of 'beyond all reasonable doubt'. This is because they were both criminal acts until the *Suicide Act 1961* (people are still said to 'commit suicide') and can have far-reaching emotional consequences for the relatives. A verdict of suicide can also cause financial problems as it may make life insurance invalid. The Coroner can bring the following verdicts:

1. Natural causes
2. Death from industrial disease
3. Drug dependence and/or abuse
4. Want of attention at birth
5. Attempted or self-induced abortion
6. Stillbirth
7. Accidental death or misadventure (arising from the consequences of a voluntary act)
8. Suicide
9. Lawful killing
10. Unlawful killing
11. Open – this means that there is insufficient evidence to decide how the deceased met his death and the case is left open in case further evidence appears.

The phrase 'aggravated by self-neglect or lack of care' can be added to the first four verdicts if appropriate and this may have implications for any healthcare professional involved. If the inquest shows that something needs to be done to prevent a recurrence, the Coroner can draw attention to it publicly and inform the relevant authority. The Coroner's decisions are subject to judicial review in the High Court but this must be requested within 3 months of the conclusion of the inquest.

The Coroner is also responsible for establishing the rightful ownership of any booty found in his district (e.g. buried treasure or the cargo of wrecked ships). This is known as establishment of 'treasure trove'.

DEATH CERTIFICATION IN SCOTLAND

Under the *Registration of Births, Deaths and Marriages (Scotland) Act 1965*, a doctor has a duty to complete a Medical Certificate of Cause of Death if he attended the deceased during the last illness. However, unlike England and Wales, the time limit is 28 days, not 14, and if the deceased did not see a doctor during that time, any doctor who knows the cause of death may complete the certificate. The death must be registered within 8 days.

The Scottish equivalent of the Coroner is the Procurator Fiscal, whose jurisdiction is the same as that of the Sheriff in whose court he appears (see Ch. 1). There are six regional Procurators Fiscal and 48 Procurator Fiscal offices, one for each Sheriff Court district. If the death is reportable, the doctor should not complete the certificate until given leave by the Fiscal. The Fiscal has a statutory duty to investigate the deaths shown in the box opposite.

The investigation is done in private and may involve:

- interviewing the relatives or other witnesses (this is usually done on his behalf by the police). This is called 'pre-cognition' and is not under oath
- calling for a further medical report. For deaths outside hospital and the usual residence of the deceased, the Forensic Medical Examiner may be required to externally examine the body to confirm death and whether or not

---

Deaths that must be investigated by the Procurator Fiscal

- Of uncertain cause
- Accidental including vehicle, train or aeroplane accidents
- Industrial including accidents, poisoning or disease
- Following abortion or attempted abortion
- Under anaesthetic
- Possibly arising from defects in medicinal products
- As a result of neglect
- Foster children
- Neonatal
- Suffocation in children, including overlaying
- Poisoning
- Food poisoning and infectious disease
- In prison or police custody
- People of no fixed abode
- Drowning
- Fire, scalding and explosion
- Suicide
- Any other violent, sudden or unexplained death

---

there are any suspicious circumstances
- ordering a post mortem, of which there are four types:
    - *Two-doctor* – where there are suspicious circumstances
    - *One-doctor* – for probable suicides, accidental or natural deaths
    - *External examination only* ('view and grant') at the discretion of the pathologist – for probable natural deaths

— *View and grant preferred* – for cases where the relatives have a strong objection to a post mortem but this is rarely used.

If the death occurred in custody or as a result of an industrial accident or it appears to the Lord Advocate that there is public interest in the case, the Fiscal is obliged by the *Fatal Accidents and Sudden Deaths Inquiry (Scotland) Act 1976* to hold a Fatal Accident Inquiry (FAI). Note that there is no routine public inquest as in the Coroner system.

APPEARING AT A FATAL ACCIDENT INQUIRY

The conduct of a FAI is very similar to the Coroner's inquest in England (see above). It is also inquisitorial and is held in public before the Sheriff without a jury, with the Fiscal leading the evidence, before questions from anyone with a 'proper interest'. The Fiscal calls the witnesses and informs any interested parties. At the conclusion of the Inquiry, the Sheriff issues a determination, which is not admissible in other courts and must set out:

- where and when the death and any accident leading to it occurred
- the cause(s) of death
- the reasonable precautions (if any) that may have prevented the death
- the defects (if any) that may have contributed to the death
- any other facts relevant to the circumstances of the death.

Note that the Sheriff does not have the range of verdicts available to the Coroner.

DEATH CERTIFICATION IN NORTHERN IRELAND

The Coroner system in Northern Ireland is similar to that of England and Wales but the relevant statute is the *Coroner's Act (Northern Ireland) 1959* and there are some differences:

- As for Scotland, the doctor can complete the Medical Certificate of Cause of Death if he saw the deceased up to 28 days prior to death.
- Both the doctor and the Registrar have a statutory duty to refer reportable deaths to the Coroner and the doctor must not complete a certificate in such cases.
- Coroners are appointed by the Lord Chancellor and they must be legally qualified. Their jurisdictions are more limited as the death must occur or the body must be found within their district.
- In jury cases, Coroners in England and Wales can accept a majority verdict, but in Northern Ireland it must be unanimous.

POST MORTEMS AND REMOVAL OF TISSUE

In deaths from natural causes, there is no legal obligation for a post mortem but it may be requested in clinical interest to establish the extent of the disease or to look for other pathology. Under the *Human Tissue Acts 1961 and 1962,* authority for hospital post mortems must come from the 'person lawfully in possession of the body', which is the Trust until the body is claimed by the next of kin or the executor(s). Permission can only be given if there is no reason to believe that either the relatives or the dead person would have objected to a post mortem. Currently, relatives are asked to confirm their lack of objection to a post mortem and to the removal of limited amounts of tissue for teaching, research and therapeutic purposes. The latter part can be deleted but the revelation that organs from dead children had been retained at Alder Hey Hospital without the permission of the parents has led to calls for the *Human Tissue Act 1961* to be amended. Relatives would then have to give informed consent to the retention of organs. In Coroners' cases, the authority for the post mortem is given by a Coroner's Order and the consent of the relatives is not required, although they are entitled to be represented at the examination by a doctor. The Coroner cannot authorize the retention of tissue for research purposes and this also applies for the Fiscal.

The legal status of tissue removed at operations (e.g. following a mastectomy) or a blood sample remains unclear. In the past, excess tissue has been used for research, drug testing and therapeutic uses (e.g. bone grafts) but it has now been argued that the donor should give informed consent prior to any use.

DISPOSAL ARRANGEMENTS

Under the *Births and Deaths Registration Act 1926,* an undertaker can only dispose of a body with either a disposal certificate from the Registrar or an Order for Burial (Form 101) from the Coroner. He must also inform the Registrar once the burial has taken place. If the relatives wish to take the body abroad for disposal or bury it at sea, they must obtain an Out of England Order from the Coroner, even if the death was from natural causes. This is because there is a loss of potential medicolegal evidence. For burials at sea, they must also notify the District Inspector of Fisheries.

There are also very strict controls over cremations. Under the Cremation Regulations, the following forms must be completed:

A. This is the application for cremation, signed by a relative or executor.

B. This is completed by the attending doctor who must have seen the body after death and he is paid a fee.

C. This is completed by a doctor of 5 or more years' full registration, who must see the body after death and question the doctor who signed Form B. He must not have been involved in the care of or be related to the deceased and he must have no known pecuniary interest. He must not be in partnership with the other doctor or related to him. He also receives a fee. This form is not necessary if the deceased died in hospital and a post mortem was performed.

D. This is issued after a post mortem requested by the medical referee of the crematorium.

E. This is issued by the Coroner and replaces forms B and C. It can be issued with or without an inquest but the cremation of people who died abroad requires authority from the Secretary of State. The Scottish equivalent is Form E(1).

F. This is the authority to cremate a body from the medical referee of the crematorium.

G. This is completed by the crematorium superintendent after the cremation.

H. This is used where the body has been used for anatomical examination under the *Anatomy Act 1984*.

Note that the medical forms ask whether or not a pacemaker has been fitted and if it has been removed. This is because they can explode during cremation. There is some doubt as to who should remove them and currently this is done by the pathologist at post mortem or by any doctor or even the embalmer or funeral director if there is no post mortem.

In Scotland, cremations can only take place once the crematorium superintendent has received Form 14, which acknowledges that the death has been registered.

Reference
1. Rutty GN, Duerden RM, Carter N, Clark JC. Are Coroners' necropsies necessary? A prospective study examining whether a 'view and grant' system of death certification could be introduced into England and Wales. J Clin Pathol 2001; 54(4): 279–284

Further reading
British Medical Association. Confirmation and certification of death. Guidelines for general practitioners in England and Wales. General practitioner committee. London: BMA, 1999
Knight B. Forensic pathology, 2nd edn. London: Arnold, 1996

Useful websites
The Coroner system:
www.homeoffice.gov.uk/ccpd/Coroner
The Procurator Fiscal system:
www.procuratorfiscal.gov.uk

CHAPTER 12

BRAIN STEM DEATH AND ORGAN DONATION

INTRODUCTION

If the brain stem is irreversibly damaged, the centres that control breathing and circulation fail and the patient dies. This is known as 'brain stem death' (BSD) and is the point at which mechanical life support should be discontinued and retrieval of organs for transplantation considered. This chapter describes the criteria that must be satisfied in order to make a diagnosis of BSD and the tests that must be performed. It further discusses the issues surrounding organ retrieval and transplantation.

DEFINITION OF DEATH

There is no statutory definition of death in the United Kingdom but it can be regarded as 'irreversible loss of the capacity for consciousness, combined with irreversible loss of the capacity to breathe'.[1] This is the clinical state that follows BSD so BSD equates with the death of the patient.

MAKING THE DIAGNOSIS OF BSD

The procedure for the diagnosis and management of BSD is outlined in Figure 12.1.

IDENTIFICATION AND CAUSE OF COMA

BSD should only be considered where there is no doubt that the patient's condition is due to irremediable brain damage of known aetiology. It must not be confused with the problems relating to the diagnosis and management of permanent vegetative state (PVS) (see Ch. 13). BSD may be diagnosed within hours (e.g. following a severe head injury) but it may take much longer (e.g. a patient who has suffered an indefinite period of cerebral hypoxia following a cardiac arrest). Other investigations such as a CT scan may be necessary to confirm the aetiology.

EXCLUSION OF OTHER CAUSES OF COMA

Hypothermia
This can occur as a consequence but it may also be the primary cause of loss of consciousness, so it is recommended that the core body temperature should be at least 35°C when the BSD tests are done.

Drugs
Those commonly used in intensive

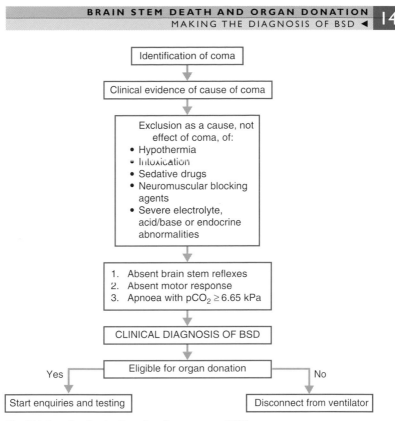

Fig. 12.1 Procedure for the diagnosis and management of BSD

care units, such as benzodiazepines or opiates, can be cumulative and have prolonged action, particularly where the patient is hypothermic or is in renal or hepatic failure. These drugs must be stopped prior to the diagnosis being made. If the patient has no spontaneous respiration but received neuromuscular blocking agents, then the persisting effects of these drugs must be excluded by either attempting to elicit the deep tendon reflexes or by demonstrating

adequate neuromuscular conduction using a nerve stimulator.

Circulatory, metabolic and electrolyte imbalances
Some disturbances, such as arrhythmias, diabetes insipidus and hypernatraemia, may be a consequence of BSD but all potentially reversible disturbances should be excluded as the cause of the coma prior to making the diagnosis.

BSD TESTS

BSD tests should be performed:

- by at least two doctors:
  - who have been registered for 5 or more years
  - who are competent in the field
  - who are not members of the transplant team
  - at least one of whom is a consultant
- on two occasions by the two doctors – either separately or together – to reduce the risk of observer error and to confirm the irreversibility of the loss of the reflexes. There is no recommended set time period between the two sets of tests as this depends on the primary pathology and the state of the patient but it should be adequate to reassure those concerned. A minimum of 2 hours has been suggested, although in France there must be 24 hours between the two sets of tests
- on the first occasion when the patient has been observed to have fixed pupils and a complete absence of cranial nerve reflex responses for at least 4 hours.

> **Note**
>
> The *legal* time of death is when the first tests indicate BSD, even though death is not *pronounced* until after the second set of tests is completed.

CLINICAL CRITERIA

The clinical criteria for BSD were established by the Conference of Colleges between 1976 and 1981[2] and are as follows:

1. *Absent brain stem reflexes* – note that it may be impossible to test all the reflexes in the presence of severe head and facial injuries. The tests shown in Table 12.1 are used to establish loss of the corresponding brain stem reflex.
2. *Absent motor responses* – no motor responses within the cranial nerve distribution can be elicited by adequate stimulation of any somatic area and there is no limb response to supraorbital pressure. Note that facial grimacing and spinal reflex movements of the limbs and torso may occur after. BSD has been established and this may need to be explained to the relatives.
3. *Apnoea with $pCO_2 \geq 6.65$ kPa* – the patient does not try to breathe once the ventilator has been disconnected and the threshold arterial pCO_2 for respiratory stimulation of 6.65 kPa has been reached. The preferred method is to ventilate the patient with 100% O_2 for 10 minutes, then with 5% CO_2 for 5 minutes. The ventilator should then be disconnected for 10 minutes and O_2 given at 8 l/min through a tracheal catheter to avoid hypoxia. The pCO_2 should be checked by measurement of the arterial blood gases but note that patients with

TABLE 12.1 Tests to establish brain stem reflexes

Reflex	Test	Reflex absent
Pupillary	Shine a *bright* light into each eye separately and observe for at least 1 minute	Pupils are fixed and do not constrict to light
Corneal	Lightly touch cornea with cotton wool, taking care not to damage it	Eye does not blink
Vestibulo-ocular (caloric)	Slowly inject ≥ 50 ml ice-cold water over 1 minute into each external auditory meatus in turn with head flexed at 30°. Check that auditory canals are clear prior to starting	Eyes do not move towards irrigated ear
Oculocephalic (doll's eye)	Turn head rapidly from one side to the other while holding the eyes open and observe eye movement (omit if there is any risk of cervical spine damage)	Eyes move with the head and do not move within the orbit

pre-existing respiratory disease may need much higher levels of pCO_2 before they are stimulated to breathe. Peripheral neurological syndromes must be excluded as a cause of the apnoea. This test should only be done after the other tests have confirmed BSD as the rise in pCO_2 provokes a rise in intracranial pressure that could endanger patients not yet dead.

The heart has been shown to stop beating a short period after fulfilment of these criteria, even if ventilation is continued.

These criteria also apply in children 2 months or older but do

Note

The criteria do not include results of tests such as CT scans or EEGs as there is no evidence at present that they assist in the determination of BSD.

not apply to those < 37 weeks. It is only rarely possible to establish BSD in babies between 37 weeks' gestation and 2 months. A Working Party of the Conference of Colleges on Organ Transplantation in Neonates recommended that organs could be removed from anencephalic infants when two doctors agree that spontaneous respiration has ceased.[3]

MANAGEMENT OF BSD

It is essential that the relatives are kept updated on the patient's condition and prognosis at all stages

and that the tests are explained. All attempts to maintain an adequate fluid intake, electrolyte balance and

---

Note

It is illegal to keep a patient on a ventilator solely to preserve organ function.[4]

---

normal blood pressure should be continued until after BSD has been diagnosed and may be continued beyond that if the patient is to be an organ donor.

Non-therapeutic (elective) ventilation is illegal as the patient does not benefit from it. It cannot be said to be in the patient's best interests, so it cannot be justified.

MANAGEMENT OF POTENTIAL ORGAN AND TISSUE DONORS

In order for a patient to become an organ donor, the following criteria must be fulfilled:

1. brain stem dead and maintained on a ventilator
2. no behavioural risk factors for HIV or hepatitis
3. no history of malignant disease except some primary brain tumours (although such patients may still donate tissue, e.g. cornea)
4. no undiagnosed systemic infection.

THE TRANSPLANT COORDINATOR

When a patient is identified as a potential donor, the transplant coordinator should be contacted as early as possible, even before formal confirmation of BSD if appropriate. However, he will not discuss the possibility of organ donation with the relatives until the medical and nursing staff have discussed the prognosis and the concept of BSD with them. The transplant coordinator will also provide the protocols to be followed and contact the United Kingdom Transplant Support Service Authority (UKTSSA) and the local transplant unit.

DONOR CARDS

If a patient carries a signed donor card or has made his wishes known in some other way (e.g. by inclusion on the NHS Organ Donation Register), then there is no legal requirement to ensure that the relatives do not object, even if the patient was a child. However, the relatives' views should be considered and if they are very opposed to the process, then it may be prudent to put their feelings first. Family refusal accounts for 30% of the failures to donate although a further 30% will offer donation before being asked. Note that neither the patient nor the relatives can impose any conditions on the use of the donated organs. An example of a current donor card is shown in Figure 12.2.

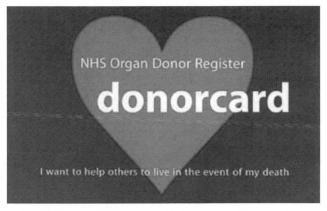

Fig. 12.2 A current donor card (©Crown copyright. Reproduced with the permission of the controller of HMSO and the Queen's Printer for Scotland)

AUTHORIZATION OF REMOVAL

If it is not known that the patient wished to donate his organs after death, then under the *Human Tissue Acts* of 1961 and 1962 (Northern Ireland), only the person who legally owns the body or his designate can authorize the removal of tissues or organs. If the body is in an NHS hospital, then the legal owner is the person with control and management of the hospital or NHS Trust until it is claimed by the person who has the right to possession of it for the purposes of disposal. This is usually the executor(s) of the will or the next of kin but may be either the Coroner or Procurator Fiscal if the death was not obviously due to natural causes. The NHS Trust can designate a person to act on its behalf and that person is usually the consultant in charge of the patient. Authorization may be given orally, but only after it has been established by 'reasonable enquiry' that:

1. the deceased had no objections to being used as an organ donor
2. the relatives do not object to the process
3. there are no religious obstacles.

Note that 'reasonable enquiry' is not defined in the *Human Tissue Act*. It is important to keep detailed, contemporaneous notes of all enquiries made and if, as recommended, the relatives are asked to sign a form, the wording should be 'lack of objection', rather than 'consent'. The person who approaches the relatives with the idea of organ donation can be a doctor, nurse, the chaplain or the transplant coordinator but it must be done with sensitivity and preferably face-to-face. If it is not practical to ask the relatives (e.g. young children) or they cannot be traced, then authorization can still be given but the situation must be carefully recorded in the transplantation checklist. Note that there is no provision in the *Human Tissue Act 1961* for penalties if tissue is taken without authorization. If there may be a need for a Coroner's post mortem, then consent must be obtained from the Coroner or Procurator Fiscal (see Ch. 11).

PAYMENT FOR ORGANS

It is a criminal offence under the *Human Organ Transplants Act 1989* to make or receive a payment in return for supplying an organ for transplantation from a dead or living person. It is also an offence to arrange such a payment or advertise for donors with the promise of remuneration. Note that 'payment' does not include the costs of removing, transporting or preserving an organ, nor loss of earnings or reasonable expenses paid to a living donor.

UKTSSA

UKTSSA (United Kingdom Transplant Support Service Authority) is a special health authority that has the following functions:

1. Matching, allocating and distributing organs for transplant.
2. Maintenance of the NHS Organ Donor Register, which contains the details of people willing to donate some or all of their organs.
3. Maintenance of the National Transplant Database, which contains details of all potential organ recipients in the UK and the Republic of Ireland.
4. Liaison with the transplant centres.
5. Liaison with the transplant coordinators.

RETRIEVAL OF ORGANS AND TISSUE

Once BSD has been confirmed and authorization given for organ removal, the transplant coordinator will contact the UKTSSA and the local transplant team. He will also organize the practical issues such as theatre time and the retrieval team and also any relevant screening tests. Malignant disease must also be excluded where possible although this is less important for certain types of tissue (e.g. corneal).

Under the *Human Tissue Act 1961*, the retrieval surgeon must personally inspect the body and the results of any tests and be satisfied that the potential donor is dead. Organ retrieval can start before the virology and bacteriology results are available but the organs cannot be transplanted until they are pronounced clear of infection. The tissues detailed in Table 12.2 can be retrieved and stored for long periods following circulatory arrest.

TABLE 12.2 Tissue storage

Tissue	Time limit (hours)
Cornea	24
Skin	48
Bone	48
Heart valves	72

ORGAN SUPPLY AND DEMAND

Demand for organs continues to outstrip the supply. For example, 112 lung transplants were performed in the UK in 1999 but there are currently over 200 patients on the waiting list. The limited supply of organs has led to rationing and consideration of measures to increase the number of organs available.

RATIONING

Rationing presents a serious ethical problem, as it is difficult to decide what parameters should be used and where the limit should lie. For example, any age limit is likely to be very arbitrary and while a physically fit patient is more likely to survive the operation, it may provide a sicker patient with their only chance of survival.

MEASURES TO INCREASE THE NUMBER OF ORGANS AVAILABLE

The following four options have been considered and present their own unique ethical dilemmas.

Opt-out system of organ donation

It has been proposed that every dying patient be regarded as a potential organ donor unless he has made his objection known. This system is practised in Austria, Belgium, France and Spain and has resulted in a sustained increase in the number of donors but it places a moral pressure on the public to participate. The British Organ Donor Society (BODY) support the use of 'presumed consent with family agreement' as this is already allowed within the *Human Tissue Act 1961* so would not require a change in the law. This would mean that staff could presume that the patient would have given consent and the family are asked to agree to organ donation, rather than have to give permission.

Living donors

This is now accepted practice for some types of transplant (e.g. bone marrow); in America, over 30% of kidney transplants come from living donors. The *Human Organ Transplants Act 1989* makes it illegal to remove an organ from a living person or to then transplant it, unless the donor and recipient are genetically related. However, the *Human Organ Transplants (Unrelated Persons) Regulations 1989* established the Unrelated Live Transplant Regulatory Authority (ULTRA), which allows, in exceptional circumstances, transplantation of organs from unrelated donors (e.g. spouses). ULTRA ensures that there is no financial inducement or coercion being applied to the donor but these regulations do not apply in cases where the donor and recipient are genetically related. Concerns have been expressed that the potential donor may suffer emotional blackmail, especially where the donor is a sibling and may be a young child.

Xenotransplantation

This is defined as the transfer of viable cells, tissues or organs between species. Some tissues (e.g. porcine heart valves and insulin) are already in common use but the transplantation of whole organs is still in the early stages. The animal of choice is the pig, which breeds quickly with large litters, has organs of equivalent size and can be both genetically modified and reared in a pathogen-free environment. However, there are numerous technical difficulties and the risk of infection with foreign pathogens in a patient who has been immunocompromised to prevent graft rejection cannot be ignored. There is also the obvious dilemma as to whether it is morally acceptable to sacrifice an animal to save a human. Xenotransplantation in the UK is regulated by the UK Xenotransplantation Interim Regulatory Authority (UKXIRA).

Foetal tissue

Experimental work has already been done on the use of foetal pancreas as a treatment for diabetes, and neural cells for Parkinson's disease, with varying degrees of success. The procedures raise several ethical issues, including the source of the foetal tissue – whether from spontaneous or induced abortions – and whether or not the mother should be told of the intended use.

DONATING A BODY TO BE USED FOR MEDICAL TEACHING PURPOSES

The deceased will normally have made advance arrangements to donate his body, so a written statement should be amongst his papers. Factors to be considered by the medical school prior to accepting the body include place and cause of death, the condition of the body and the demand for bodies. Bodies are usually refused if there has been a post mortem or if organs other than the corneas have been removed. Bodies may be kept for teaching purposes for up to 3 years and are then cremated or buried at a special memorial service with the costs borne by the medical school.

References

1. Department of Health. A code of practice for the diagnosis of brain stem death. London: DoH, 1998
2. Criteria for the diagnosis of brain stem death. J R Col Phys 1995; 21: 381–382
3. Working party on organ transplantation in neonates. Conference of Medical Colleges and Faculties of the United Kingdom. London: DHSS, 1988
4. Identification of potential donors of organs for transplantation. HSG (94)41 NHS Executive; Interventional ventilation and organ transplantation DGM 94(116) Welsh Office; Elective ventilation NHS MEL(1994) The Scottish Office

Useful websites

www.uktransplant.org.uk
British Organ Donor Society
(BODY): www.argonet.co.uk/body

CHAPTER 13

EUTHANASIA, WITHDRAWAL OF TREATMENT AND ADVANCE DIRECTIVES

INTRODUCTION

There has been much confusion over the terms 'euthanasia' and 'withdrawing or withholding treatment' but the simplest distinction that can be made is that euthanasia involves an active intervention to end life whereas withdrawal of treatment means not attempting to prolong life. Until recently, most countries believed that passive euthanasia, i.e. letting a patient die, is acceptable whereas an active euthanasia of killing is not. There now seems to be a shift from refusal of treatment to a request for aid to die. Healthcare professionals currently have a moral and legal obligation to act upon a valid Advance Directive that refuses treatment. If valid requests for aid to die become legal as in Oregon, then healthcare professionals may find themselves facing that same obligation to arrange a patient's death.

EUTHANASIA

INTRODUCTION

Euthanasia has been defined as 'procuring a painless and easy death' and its legalisation is the subject of much heated discussion. It has furious opposition but also fervent supporters and has stimulated many legal, ethical, moral and religious debates.

There are four forms of euthanasia:

- *Voluntary active* – a competent adult asks a third party to help him to die
- *Voluntary passive* – a competent adult dies following withdrawal of treatment at his request
- *Involuntary passive* – treatment is withdrawn or withheld from an incompetent patient, e.g. unconscious or comatose
- *involuntary active* – this is murder!

In *physician-assisted suicide*, a doctor prescribes a lethal drug but it is either administered by the patient himself or by a third party, such as a nurse or relative. Studies have shown that doctors prefer physician-assisted suicide as it confers a more passive role but complications during administration may result in the doctor giving the drug and hence performing euthanasia.

HISTORY

Existing laws allow terminally ill people to request the removal of life-sustaining medical interventions and to receive palliative drugs that may hasten death. In 1996, an Appeals Court in America held that those who wish to hasten their death but are not dependent on life-sustaining technology are unequally treated and therefore physician-assisted suicide should be legally available. The following year, the Supreme Court of the United States ruled that 'the right to commit suicide with another's assistance' was not a constitutional right and not the same as the right to refuse treatment. However, it also said that physician-assisted suicide was not unconstitutional and that each State could decide the issue on an individual basis.

LEGAL POSITION

The only American State that has legalized physician-assisted suicide so far is Oregon, which passed the *Death with Dignity Act* in 1994. This allows doctors to prescribe but not administer lethal drugs on written request to competent patients with less than 6 months to live. Two witnesses must sign the request and at least two doctors must agree that the patient is likely to die within 6 months. The Act protects the doctor from future litigation or disciplinary procedures. In contrast, 34 States, including Washington, have statutes that explicitly make assisted suicide a criminal act.

In 1996, the Northern Territory of Australia passed the *Rights of the Terminally Ill Act*, which legalized voluntary euthanasia. Four Australians used it to die before it was overturned by the Federal Parliament in 1997.

In Holland, euthanasia and assisted suicide are still criminal acts but a Bill passed in April 2001 means that a physician who helps a patient to die but complies with the

following two conditions will be exempt from punishment:

1. He must practise due care as set out in the *Termination of Life on Request and Assisted Suicide (Review) Act 2002*. This is judged by a regional review committee and if they believe due care was not practised, then a report is sent by the Public Prosecutor for consideration of criminal proceedings.
2. He must report the cause of death as euthanasia to the Coroner in accordance with the *Burial and Cremation Act 1991*.

The 'due care' requirements include:

- The request be voluntary and well-considered
- The condition be terminal and the pain unbearable
- At least one other doctor agrees.

Both assisted suicide and euthanasia are illegal in the United Kingdom and are opposed by both the Royal College of Nursing and the British Medical Association. However, they are practised under the doctrine of 'double effect', which differentiates between the actions of the healthcare professional where death is either foreseen or intended. A healthcare professional who gives a large dose of morphine knows that the patient may die through respiratory depression but he considers it justifiable as the patient will also benefit from the pain relief, i.e. there is a 'double effect'. However, if he deliberately gives a large dose of potassium chloride, his only intention can be to cause the death of that patient, as there is no therapeutic value. The outcome is the same but ethically and legally the two situations are very different.

Healthcare professionals in the United Kingdom can legally give unlimited amounts of pain relief so long as this is seen to be in the 'best interests' of the patient, even if the patient's life is shortened as a result. Deliberate administration of a lethal drug with no therapeutic benefit on the other hand is murder, although the courts may be lenient. In 1992, Dr Cox[1] gave a lethal dose of potassium chloride with consent to a patient with intractable pain who said that she wanted to die. He was convicted of attempted murder but received only a suspended sentence and he was reinstated at work.

It has been suggested that if euthanasia was legalized, then there would be greater safeguards on its performance while others fear that legalisation would allow uninhibited involuntary euthanasia. Data from Oregon and the Netherlands do not support either argument.

WITHDRAWAL OF TREATMENT

PERMANENT VEGETATIVE STATE (PVS)

PVS is distinct from brain stem death (see Ch. 12) in that the brain stem still functions while the cortex does not. This means that the patient can breathe unaided and the autonomic nervous system works but he cannot see, hear, speak, feel pain or move voluntarily although he still has reflex movement. It is diagnosed when the following criteria have been satisfied:[2]

1. The patient shows no evidence of awareness of self or environment
2. There is brain damage, usually of known cause, consistent with the diagnosis
3. There are no reversible causes present
4. At least 6 (and usually 12) months have passed since the onset.

However, the diagnosis of PVS cannot be absolutely certain, data on prognosis are limited and there is no standard test of awareness so there are many ethical issues surrounding the withdrawal of treatment.

PRINCIPLES OF WITHDRAWAL OF TREATMENT

- Healthcare professionals draw a distinction between withdrawing and withholding treatment but most courts do not.
- If there is a possibility that the patient will receive benefit from the treatment, then it should be continued and effective palliation should never be withdrawn.
- The decision to stop treatment must be on the basis that to continue would be futile, not because the patient has become incompetent, and it should never be denied solely on the basis of cost.

- The autonomy of the patient must be respected and basic care and nutrition should continue, although tube feeding may be regarded as a treatment and can be stopped where there is no chance of recovery.
- Communication with the relatives is vital and although the final decision should be made by the doctors, it is advisable to seek their agreement.
- At present, guidance from the High Court should *always* be sought before withholding life-prolonging treatment.

LEGAL POSITION

The most famous case in the debate about withdrawal of treatment was that of *Airedale NHS Trust v Bland 1992/3*.[3] In this case, Anthony Bland was left in PVS after being crushed in the Hillsborough Football Stadium disaster of April 1989. The Trust and the family asked the court if it would be lawful to discontinue artificial life support of hydration and nutrition and any further medical treatment as the situation was hopeless and cessation would lead to his death. The court agreed but the Official Solicitor appealed on behalf of Anthony and this was upheld in the Court of Appeal. The Trust and the family appealed to the House of Lords where it was decided that the principle of sanctity of life is not absolute and does not compel a doctor to feed a patient against his will or keep a terminally ill patient alive against his wishes. There is just as much duty to discontinue as to continue treatment and the decision must be based on what the patient would have wished had he been able to decide. The court ruled that nasogastric feeding was a treatment and also that a decision to withhold a life-sustaining treatment would not *necessarily* lead to criminal liability. Gastrostomy feeding has now been withdrawn from about 20 people diagnosed as being in PVS in the UK and, in each case, the High Court gave permission to stop feeding on the basis that the patient would not benefit from continued treatment. It did not decree that treatment *had* to stop.

ADVANCE DIRECTIVES

INTRODUCTION

An Advance Directive is a statement made by a mentally competent adult that gives instructions about how he would wish to be treated in the event of any future loss of mental capacity. It is also known as a 'living will'. An Advance Directive may be seen as a method of extending a person's autonomy by allowing him to make or convey decisions from which he would otherwise have been excluded on the basis of incapacity. Competence, capacity and methods of assessment are discussed in Chapter 5.

HISTORY

Advance Directives were introduced in America in 1967. American healthcare is predominantly private and resource driven so doctors tend to be far more interventional than those in the United Kingdom. Advance Directives were proposed as a method of restricting the number of invasive procedures being imposed on patients who did not want them. The Voluntary Euthanasia Society followed suit in the United Kingdom in the early 1970s but with a greater emphasis on patient choice. Initially, the close association of Advance Directives with the euthanasia movements limited their use but they became more widely accepted once they were seen as a method of exercising autonomy rather than simply the right to die. The first statutory support came in the *Natural Death Act of California* in 1976 and now most American States have a statutory obligation to allow Advance Directives. There is also federal legislation in the form of the *Patient Self-Determination Act 1991,* which compels hospitals and nursing homes to give patients the opportunity to make an Advance Directive at the time of admission. However, in a national survey in 1996, only 10% of Americans had made an Advance Directive with a definite racial, cultural and educational bias.[4]

LEGAL POSITION

Although many States of America, Canada and Australia now have specific legislation that requires healthcare professionals to adhere to valid Advance Directives, the legal position in the United Kingdom remains unclear. In 1993, a patient's advance refusal of treatment became legally binding under common law (see Ch. 1) with the ruling that a schizophrenic inpatient of Broadmoor could refuse amputation of his gangrenous leg then and at any time in the future, even if he became incompetent.[5] In the same year, in the case of Bland (see above), the judges stated that if he had made an Advance Directive prior to his injury, then it would have been legally binding.

In 1995, the Law Commission endorsed 'advance statements about health' and recommended legislation. It further recommended that statute law should clearly stipulate how competent adults could control their future care. Later that year a code of practice for Advance Directives was published jointly by the British Medical Association and the Royal Colleges of Nursing, Physicians and General Practitioners.[6] In 1999, the NHS Executive issued guidance on withholding consent to treatment[7] and this was closely followed by guidance from the General Medical Council on the legal position of Advance Directives.[8] In 2000, a questionnaire survey of NHS trusts showed that only about 25% had developed or intended to develop policies on Advance Directives with only a few providing help or information to patients. This led the authors to call for the development of national guidelines on Advance Directives.[9]

The Government has since stated that, as a general point of law, all adults have the right to consent to or refuse medical treatment (see Ch. 5), and that Advance Directives are a means by which patients can continue that right when they are no longer able to make that decision. There are currently no plans to introduce guidelines or legislation to govern Advance Directives and there is no legal provision to allow the nomination of a proxy decision maker. It has been suggested that if Advance Directives were legalized, then healthcare professionals would be more likely to acquaint themselves with them. An Advance Directive will have legal standing if the following conditions are met:

Conditions relating to an Advance Directive

1. The author was mentally competent, over 18 and not under any duress at the time of completion
2. The author was fully informed about the nature and possible consequences of an Advance Directive at the time of completion
3. The situations to which the Advance Directive applies are clearly stated and now apply
4. The Advance Directive has not been amended or revoked
5. The author is now incompetent to make his own decision
6. The Advance Directive refuses certain treatments or specifies the level of deterioration at which active treatment should cease

---

TYPES

There are many different types of Advance Directive but they do not have to be written in any particular format and can be verbal. The Voluntary Euthanasia Society provides a 'living will' form in .pdf format that can be downloaded from its website, along with instructions on its use (Fig. 13.1).

Some authors have proposed that the term 'Advance Directive' implies that the statement specifically requests treatments and have suggested that it might be more appropriate to call them 'Advance Refusals' but this does seem to be overpedantic. 'Disease-specific' Advance Directives have also been proposed that list the interventions which may be considered in different illnesses. The patient can then refuse specific treatments, rather than all. In America, under the Surrogacy Acts, there is a further distinction that allows for the nomination of one or more people to make decisions on behalf of the signatory, in which case the form is called an 'Enduring Power of Attorney for Healthcare'.

THE SCOPE OF ADVANCE DIRECTIVES

Note

A patient can legally refuse treatment but cannot request it.

The Law Commission argued that Advance Directives (or refusals) should:

LIVING WILL DIRECTIVE

My full name . . . .

My full address . . . .

. . . .

. . . .

My postcode. . . . .   My phone number. . . . .

My date of birth . . . .

GP's name. . . . .

GP's address. . . . .

. . . .

. . . .

GP's telephone number . . . .

I have discussed the contents of this form with my GP ☐ Yes   ☐ No

I have discussed the contents with another health professional mentioned below
☐ Yes   ☐ No   . . . .

If it is the opinion of two independent doctors that there is no reasonable prospect of my recovery from severe physical illness, or from impairment expected to cause me severe distress or render me incapable of rational existence, then I direct that I be allowed to die and not be kept alive by artificial means such as life support systems, tube feeding, antibiotics, resuscitation or blood transfusions: any treatment which has no benefit other than a mere prolongation of my existence should be withheld or withdrawn, even if it means my life is shortened. I accept basic care however and I request aggressive palliative care, drugs or any other measures to keep me free of pain or distress, even if they shorten my life. If the time comes when I can no longer communicate, this declaration shall be taken as a testament to my wishes regarding medical care. I have made this declaration at a time when I am of sound mind and after careful consideration.

I understand that my life may be shortened by the refusals of treatment in this form.

I accept the risk that I may not be able to change my mind in the future when I am no longer able to speak for myself, and I accept the risk that improving medical technology may offer increased hope, but I personally consider the risk of unwanted treatment to be a greater risk. I want it to be known that I fear degradation and indignity far more than death. I ask my

P.T.O.

Fig. 13.1 Example of a 'living will'. (Courtesy of Chris Docker MPhil, Law & Ethics in Medicine, Director, Living Will & Values History Project, BM 718, London WCIN 3XX)

medical attendants to bear this in mind when considering what my intentions would be in any uncertain situation.

I have the following wishes about specific treatments or investigation: . . . .

. . . .

. . . .

. . . .

. . . .

My other wishes/personal statement: . . . .

. . . .

. . . .

. . . .

. . . .

I wish the following person to be consulted in the event of uncertainty about my wishes:

Person's name . . . .

Person's address . . . .

. . . .

. . . .

Person's telephone number . . . .

My Signature . . . . **Date** . . . .

Witness (name) . . . .

Signature of witness . . . .

Address of witness . . . .

Reviewed: Date: . . . . My signature . . . .

Reviewed: Date: . . . . My signature . . . .

N.B. Document remains valid unless revoked orally or in writing, but reviewing and re-affirming it at approximately three year intervals is recommended.

Health Care Workers: For further information on Living Wills, please contact the Living Will and Values History Project at BM 718 London WC1N 3XX, or the Ethics Department of the British Medical Association.

Fig. 13.1 (*Continued*) Example of a 'living will'.

- not dictate the type or amount of treatment that a patient should receive. The patient's wishes should be considered but treatment remains an ultimately clinical (and often, managerial) decision
- be made by people competent to do so: able to understand, retain and act on the information on which the refusal is based
- be presumed to be valid if signed and witnessed
- be revocable if the patient is competent to revoke them
- explicitly state the author's awareness that death might or will be the result of the refusal
- be suspended if being assessed by a court for validity
- not preclude the provision of basic care, defined as the maintenance of bodily cleanliness, relief of sustained and serious pain, and the provision of oral nutrition and hydration
- not be deliberately ignored, such action being a criminal offence.

Further, a patient cannot refuse treatment:

- that has been required by law
- if this condition would put others at risk.

There are some special circumstances:

- People younger than 18 cannot make Advance Directives but the *Children Act 1989* emphasizes that their wishes must be taken into account when deciding on their treatment if they have reached the level of 'Gillick competence' (see Ch. 5).

- A patient detained under the *Mental Health Act 1983* can make a valid Advance Directive providing that he is competent to do so but only about those treatments not specified under the terms of his detention.
- If a woman is pregnant when her Advance Directive becomes valid, then the needs of the foetus supersede compliance with it.

If an Advance Directive nominates a proxy decision maker, then that person currently has no legal right to make any decisions in England, Wales and Northern Ireland. The final decision still rests with the doctor who should act in the 'best interests' of the patient, although the doctor should be guided by the nominee. A power of attorney only relates to financial and property matters. In Scotland, people older than 16 can appoint a 'tutor-dative' under the *Adults with Incapacity (Scotland) Act 2000* who then has the authority to make medical decisions on behalf of the patient. The tutor-dative may also have the authority to refuse treatment on behalf of an incompetent patient if this can be shown to be in accordance with the patient's wishes but this has not yet been tested in court.

ADVANTAGES OF ADVANCE DIRECTIVES

- They recognize the autonomy of the patient and give him peace of mind.
- Healthcare professionals are reassured that they are providing the type of care that the patient

would have wanted without fear of possible future legal redress.

- They provide an opportunity for healthcare professionals to discuss future management with the relatives.
- They relieve the relatives of making decisions for which they do not wish to be responsible.

DISADVANTAGES OF ADVANCE DIRECTIVES

- Assessment of competence may be difficult and subject to later criticism.
- Refusal of treatment must be fully informed but it can only be valid if the facts relating to the current situation are available. Most Advance Directives are made years prior to mental incompetence, when details of the conditions specified and any possible treatments were not known.
- Advances in medical treatment may invalidate an Advance Directive by changing the situations to which it applies.
- The patient may change his mind.
- Advance Directives only cover refusal of treatment and other factors may be equally important to the patient, such as place of death.
- There is no routine provision for recording the existence and whereabouts of an Advance Directive although it has been suggested that this should be done when the patient is admitted to hospital or a nursing home.
- The healthcare professional may find it hard to accept that the

patient may prefer death, particularly if the patient is unable to speak. However, if he feels unable to follow the Advance Directive for ethical reasons, then he must transfer the care of that patient to another healthcare professional.

- Conservatism – it is easier to do something than nothing, particularly in situations when failure to treat cannot be reversed and may result in litigation.

MAKING AN ADVANCE DIRECTIVE

If you are asked to witness or help compose an Advance Directive, you should ensure that the following criteria have been met:

Criteria for the patient

1. Is competent – this must be presumed unless there is evidence to the contrary
2. Is aware of the legal standing
3. Is able to understand the implications
4. Can accurately forsee possible future circumstances in which it might apply
5. Is fully informed about his diagnosis, prognosis and possible treatments
6. Is aware of potential future advances in the treatment of his disease
7. Is aware that the Advance Directive can be revoked at any time
8. Has plans to regularly review the Advance Directive
9. Is not under any duress

Patients should be discouraged from making Advance Directives when they are acutely unwell or soon after being given a poor prognosis. They should also be told that it is their responsibility to ensure that any healthcare professional involved in their future care is made aware of the existence of the Advance Directive. Advance Directives should preferably be written on a pre-prepared form and witnessed by a doctor and/or lawyer, as this

⚠ If the Advance Directive appears to be valid, comply with the refusal of treatment. If there is *any* doubt, act in the 'best interests' of the patient and seek further advice.

makes them less likely to be challenged in court but if the patient insists on writing his own statement, then it must contain the following:

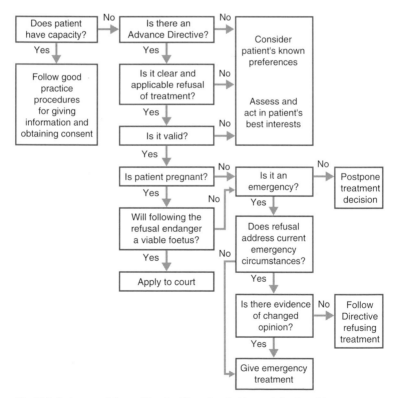

Fig. 13.2 Acting on an Advance Directive. (Reproduced with permission from *Advance Statements about Medical Treatment.* BMA, 1995.)

- Name, address and date of birth of the patient
- Name and address of his GP and/or hospital consultant
- Whether or not medical advice was sought
- Patient's signature and date
- Date of first review
- Signature of at least one witness (preferably two, including the patient's doctor or lawyer)
- A clear statement of the patients' wishes.

WHAT TO DO IF GIVEN AN ADVANCE DIRECTIVE

- Ensure that the patient is the one named in the Advance Directive and was over 18 at the time of completion.
- Examine him and assess his level of competence – he must be incompetent for the Advance Directive to come into effect.
- Ask for a second opinion.
- Contact any witnesses if possible. If his doctor was a witness, check that the patient was competent at the time and not under any duress.
- Contact any nominated proxies but ensure that they are aware that they have no legal rights.
- Check that the current situation is specified in the Advance Directive.
- Carefully document all decisions.
- Follow the flow chart shown in Figure 13.2.

References

1. *R v Cox* [1992] 12 BMLR 1
2. Wade DT. Ethical issues in diagnosis and management of patients in the permanent vegetative state. BMJ 2001; 322: 352–354
3. *Airedale NHS Trust v Bland* [1993] 1 All ER 821, (1993) 12 BMLR 64
4. Hanson LC, Rodgman E. The use of living wills at the end of life: a national study. Arch Int Med 1996; 156(9): 1018–1062
5. *Re C* [1994] 1 All ER 819, (1993) 15 BMLR 77
6. British Medical Association. Advance statements about medical and treatment. Code of practice and explanatory notes. London: BMA, 1995
7. NHS Executive. Consent to treatment; summary of legal rulings. London: NHSE, 1999 (HSC 1999/031)
8. General Medical Council. Seeking patient's consent: the ethical considerations. London: GMC, 1999
9. Diggory P, Judd M. Advance directives: questionnaire survey of NHS trusts. BMJ 2000; 320: 24–25

Further reading

British Medical Association. Withholding or withdrawing life-prolonging medical treatment. Guidance for decision making. London: BMA, 1999

Useful websites

Right To Life: www.righttolife.org.uk
Voluntary Euthanasia Society: www.ves.org.uk

CHAPTER 14

CHILD ABUSE AND THE CHILDREN ACTS

INTRODUCTION

Child abuse is perhaps one of the most distressing areas in which a healthcare professional may become involved. This chapter aims to outline the features in the history and examination of a child that should make the healthcare professional suspicious that the injuries seen may not be accidental in origin. It also covers the laws that relate to children with a detailed discussion of the *Children Acts*. It does not cover child sexual abuse but for those who would like to read more on the subject, there is an excellent chapter in *Clinical Forensic Medicine* in the Further reading list.

LEGAL ASPECTS

There are some laws that relate specifically to children, as follows.

INFANTICIDE

This is the deliberate killing of an infant under the age of 12 months, although deaths usually occur within hours or minutes of birth. It must be shown that the infant had a separate existence and that death occurred as a result of an act of either deliberate commission or omission. This may be very difficult to prove, particularly if the birth was initially concealed. The *Infanticide Act 1938* allows courts in England and Wales to take a lenient view of a mother that kills her infant while the 'balance of her mind was disturbed by reason of her not having fully recovered from the effects of giving birth to the child, or by reason of the effect of lactation consequent upon the birth of the child'. However, it is still regarded as child murder in Scotland.

STILLBIRTH

This is defined in the *Stillbirth (Definition) Act 1992* and the *Still-Births (Scotland) Act 1938* as an infant who was born after 24 weeks' gestation and never showed signs of life after being expelled from the mother. It affects 1 in 50 births and involves special certification to allow collection of statistical data on the cause of death (stillbirth certificate – see Ch. 11). Note that foetuses born before 24 weeks are not registered.

CHILD DESTRUCTION

This is the killing of a foetus in utero after 28 weeks (*Infant Life Preservation Act 1929*).

CONCEALMENT OF BIRTH

This is defined in the *Offences against the Person Act 1861 (England and Wales)* and the *Concealment of Birth (Scotland) Act 1809* as the hiding of a body to conceal the fact of birth. The cause of death, viability and whether stillborn or alive are all immaterial.

OTHER OFFENCES

Other offences that apply for all ages, and their respective sentences, are as follows:

- *Common assault* – this is threatening behaviour and commands a maximum penalty of 6 months' imprisonment or a fine
- *Battery* – this is the infliction of personal violence (penalty as for common assault)
- *Actual bodily harm (ABH)* – this is intentional assault occasioning physical injury, for example bruising (5 years)
- *Grievous bodily harm (GBH)* – this is intentional wounding resulting in a breach in the skin or GBH, for example a fracture (Life, although this is rarely given)
- *Manslaughter* (Life)
- *Murder* (Life).

DIAGNOSIS OF CHILD ABUSE

Most healthcare professionals are reluctant to make a diagnosis of child abuse for fear of 'getting it wrong'. However, there are several points in the history and examination of any child that should make the healthcare professional suspicious of non-accidental injury (NAI) (Table 14.1).

TABLE 14.1 Risk factors for child abuse

Parents or guardians	Child
Social class IV and V but can occur in all young/immature parents	Premature – extra feeding with poor response
Abused in childhood themselves	'Wrong' sex
Denied request for termination of pregnancy	Sick children
Sporadic or no antenatal attendance	Under 2 years of age
Denial of access to health visitor and social workers	Multiple births
Present co-habitee is not the father of the child	Both boys and girls
Unemployed or made redundant	First born
Further pregnancies	Any abnormality – especially learning disabilities
Drugs and/or alcohol abuse	
Illness	
No social support	

HISTORY

1. *History inconsistent with injury* – the story given must match the type of injury, e.g. a cigarette burn is not caused by a boiling cup of tea.

2. *History inconsistent with developmental milestones* – a 6-week old baby cannot 'roll off the bed'.

3. *Varying or changing explanations* – the child may give a different explanation if he is interviewed in the absence of the parents as may each parent. The story may also change as the family see different healthcare professionals.

4. *Delay in reporting the injury* – old injuries should raise suspicions unless there is a reasonable explanation for the delay such as a holiday abroad or that the child has been with a different carer. This is particularly important if there are multiple injuries of different ages.

5. *'Hospital hopping'* – abusive parents often take their children to different agencies, including different general practitioner surgeries in an effort to avoid the child being highlighted as a frequent attendee. They may also give different names and details.

EXAMINATION

1. *Fear of one or both parents* – abused children may appear frightened but, conversely, they may be excessively affectionate towards the parent in an effort to gain approval.

2. *Poor eye contact* – this is commonly seen in people who are not telling the truth and may involve the child and/or the carer.

3. *'Frozen awareness'* – this is a classic trait in children who have been abused over a long period, denoting a child who is either incapable or fearful of displaying any emotion.

4. *Excessive compliance with examination* – children are naturally shy and often reluctant to undress in front of strangers. Abused children are frequently overly eager to comply with any instructions given.

5. *Seeking comfort from staff* – any child who prefers to be comforted by staff rather than the carer must be examined carefully for signs of abuse.

6. *Multiple injuries of differing ages* – all children get injured accidentally and may have multiple injuries but they are usually minor and always on exposed prominent areas such as knees and elbows. However, the carer or child should be asked for explanations for any injuries seen and a note made of any previous attendances for the more serious injuries.

7. *Different types of injury* – this is particularly important if all the injuries are of a similar age.

8. *Multiple injuries from single cause* – for example cigarette burns.

TYPES OF INJURY

SURFACE INJURIES

Some surface injuries are diagnostic of child abuse, others are suspicious but must be viewed in conjunction with other signs. The following are classic injuries:

- *Black eyes* – children rarely get black eyes accidentally.
- *'Tin ear'* – this is bruising of the pinna caused by slap to the head.
- *Slap marks* – these are linear petechial marks, often in the shape of a hand and commonly seen on the face.
- *Torn frenulum in babies* – this is caused by a bottle being forced into the mouth, usually in an attempt to stop the baby crying.
- *Bruising around mouth* – this is indicative of smothering; again it is usually done in an attempt to silence the child.
- *Subcomunctival haemorrhages* – these are also indicative of smothering and also attempted strangulation and shaking.
- *Bald patches* – from hair pulling.

BRUISES

All children (and many adults) have bruises. They are often multiple but the following should raise suspicions of a non-accidental origin:

- *Spot bruises* (Fig. 14.1) – these suggest pinch and fingertip marks. They are most commonly found on the limbs, chest and abdomen.

- *Knuckle punches* (Fig. 14.2) – these are rows of three or four round bruises.
- *Characteristic patterns* – some bruises have distinctive shapes that pertain to the implement used, e.g. tramline bruising from sticks (Fig. 14.3); belt buckle marks.

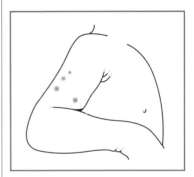

Fig. 14.1 Spot bruises on the upper arm

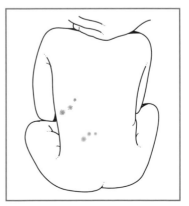

Fig. 14.2 Knuckle punches

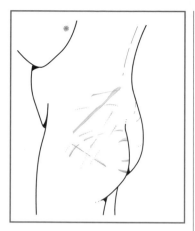

Fig. 14.3 Tramline bruising following beating with a stick

- *Bruising in inaccessible areas* – e.g. inner thighs, spine or face in babies less than 18 months old.

BITES

Bite marks are distinctive crescentic bruises, often found on the buttocks or limbs and usually multiple. It is important to distinguish adult bites from those done by children – juvenile bites are smaller with a narrower arch. It is also vital to distinguish human bites from animal ones – humans make more use of the molars so there is more bruising and less piercing of the skin.

BURNS

Children often burn themselves accidentally but 10% of abused children are burnt. Unless there is other pathology such as epilepsy, then deep burns in children are almost exclusively the result of abuse as they indicate prolonged contact with the offending object. There are certain types of burn that are characteristic of child abuse:

- *'Dipping' scalds* (Fig. 14.4) – these are scalds that are confined to the buttocks and heels, where the child has been dipped in boiling water. The story given is that the child sat down in a hot bath but if that were true, then the child would also have scalds to the top of the feet and it is unlikely that the child would then have sat down.
- *Cigarette burns* (Fig. 14.5) – these are circular burns that are often full thickness. They are usually multiple and often in exposed areas.
- *Friction burns* – these indicate that the child has been dragged or tied up.
- *Burns in non-exposed areas or multiple burns from same source* – e.g. from a domestic iron.

SKELETAL

Unlike accidental injuries, deliberate skeletal injuries usually occur as a result of torsion, angulation or traction rather than direct impact. Abused children often have multiple fractures of varying ages which occur in sites that are rarely injured accidentally (e.g. limbs in non-walking babies and ribs). Rib fractures in a child under 5 years are pathognomonic of abuse by squeezing and the chest X-ray may show the classic 'string of beads' appearance of the healing calluses.

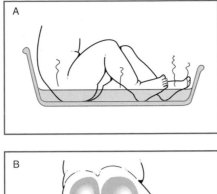

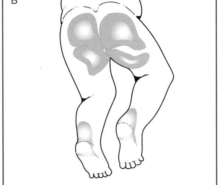

Fig. 14.4 Dipping scalds

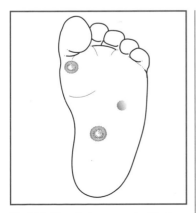

Fig. 14.5 Cigarette burns on sole of foot

Metaphyseal chipping suggests shaking and areas of periosteal calcification denote 'near fractures', i.e. that a force has been applied but that it was not sufficient to actually break the bone. Other skeletal injuries such as spiral diaphyseal and epiphyseal fractures can occur accidentally but are much more common in abused children.

HEAD INJURIES

Head injuries are the commonest cause of death from abuse and over 95% of serious head injuries in children under 1 year are due to abuse. They range from bruises, abrasions and lacerations to more serious intracranial bleeds such as subdural haematomas and subarachnoid haemorrhages. Abused children also have a higher incidence of cerebral contusions, which are associated with learning disabilities. If there are associated retinal haemorrhages, then this indicates a shaking component to the abuse (see below). Skull fractures occur most commonly in the occipitoparietal area whatever the cause, but it must be remembered that an infant must fall at least 4 feet onto a hard surface to cause a skull fracture and diffuse brain injury.[1] This means that a story that the child with a skull fracture 'rolled off the bed' is unlikely to be true.

VISCERAL INJURIES

The second most common cause of death from NAI is a ruptured liver. Other visceral injuries seen are ruptured spleen, pancreas and torn bowel – particularly the duodenum at its point of attachment. All these injuries require a huge amount of blunt force and cannot be explained by 'he fell off my lap'.

SHAKEN BABY SYNDROME

Shaken baby syndrome (SBS) was first proposed by Caffey in 1946. It describes a clinical and pathological entity characterized by retinal and subdural and/or subarachnoid haemorrhages with minimal or absent signs of external trauma. It achieved worldwide recognition in the case of Louise Woodward who was convicted of shaking 8-month old Matthew Eappen to death in 1997 despite both sides agreeing that Matthew showed signs of direct head trauma so was, by definition, not a victim of SBS.

SBS is thought to be caused by the whiplash action of the child's relatively heavy head in association with weak neck muscles, resulting in an acceleration–deceleration force sufficient to tear the bridging veins. The infant head is made further susceptible to this type of injury by an immature, partially membranous skull, a relatively large subarachnoid space and a soft immature brain. However, the original studies had no scientific basis and were mainly the result of hearsay. It now seems unlikely that such injuries can occur without some form of impact.

MUNCHAUSEN SYNDROME BY PROXY

This is an uncommon form of abuse but it carries a high morbidity and mortality with a high incidence of reabuse. The carer, usually the mother, either deliberately makes the child ill or fabricates the symptoms. The child is then subjected to a series of investigations, which often makes the situation and the eventual diagnosis even more difficult. The commonest presentations are fits, bleeding, diarrhoea, vomiting, fever and rash.

MISTAKEN DIAGNOSES

The following can mimic NAI and lead to a mistaken diagnosis:

- Vitamin and mineral deficiencies, e.g. vitamins C (scurvy) and D (rickets), copper, calcium
- Clotting abnormalities, e.g. haemophilia, von Willebrand's
- Bone disorders, e.g. osteogenesis imperfecta
- Pigment abnormalities, Mongolian spots, birth marks, striae

- Alopecia areata can mimic hair pulling
- Skin lesions, e.g. impetigo can mimic cigarette burns
- Self-inflicted injuries in older children
- Injuries inflicted by siblings or other children
- Accidental injuries.

THE CHILDREN ACT 1989

The *Children Act 1989* was first implemented in October 1991 and provided a fundamental change in child law in England and Wales. It has 108 sections and 15 schedules, with over 30 sets of rules and regulations. It is concerned with civil, not criminal law and has two fundamental principles:

1. A child is best served by staying with the family of origin without recourse to legal proceedings
2. If changes need to be made, any delay is bad for the child (section 1(2)).

   The Act makes the welfare of the child paramount. It recognizes that children have rights and that their views must be respected in the appropriate circumstances. Section 1 states that no court orders will be made unless clearly in the best interests of the child and it outlines the following checklist that a court *must* consider in determining what a child's welfare demands:

1. The ascertainable wishes of the child – note that this is the first, although not necessarily the most crucial, decision
2. Physical, emotional and educational needs
3. Likely effect of any change in circumstances

4. Age, sex, background and any other relevant characteristics
5. Any current or potential harm to the child
6. Capability of the carer to meet the needs of the child
7. The range of powers available to the court under the Act – the Act provides a choice of orders that are available to all courts and may be used in all types of proceedings.

Issues affecting a child's future

There are four main ways in which issues affecting a child's future may be brought before a court:

● *Wardship* – any individual may make a child a ward of court by issuing a summons, thereby ensuring that no decision affecting the life of the child can be made without leave of the court, for example withdrawal of treatment in a severely handicapped child. The *Children Act* restricted the powers of local authorities by not allowing them to make a child a ward of court without bringing care proceedings first.
● *Divorce proceedings*
● *Private law applications* – e.g. contact orders for estranged grandparents.
● *Care proceedings* – local authorities had extensive powers in child welfare but they were limited by the *Children Act,* which makes compulsory state intervention a last resort. A court can now only make a care order, placing a child under the supervision of the local authority if 'significant harm' can be demonstrated, this being defined as a 'deficit in or detriment to the standard of health development and well-being'. The court must also be satisfied that a care order would be in the 'best interests' of the child and *better than no order at all.* This is the 'presumption of non-intervention' and has been considered by some to be the most important provision in the Act – the concept that a care order may not necessarily be the best way to protect the child's welfare.

Orders

The Act gives all courts essentially the same powers and remedies and gives them timetables to reduce delay. It also outlines a 'menu' of orders available to the courts, including:

● *Residence order* – this replaces the custody order and defines where and with whom the child will live
● *Contact order* – this replaces the access order and defines persons with whom the child must be allowed to have contact
● *Prohibited steps order* – this stops a person with parental responsibility from making certain decisions over the child's welfare without recourse to the courts
● *Specific issues order* – this gives directions for dealing with a particular aspect of the child's care.

Parental responsibility

The Act promotes the idea of parental 'responsibility' rather than parental 'rights' and emphasizes that this responsibility continues despite divorce and when the child is in the care of a local authority, recommending the involvement of parents in child protection conferences. It defines those who have 'parental responsibility' as:

- The *mother and father* of a legitimate child, even after divorce
- The *adoptive parents* of a legally adopted child
- The *mother* of an illegitimate child although the genetic father can gain it through a parental responsibility order, agreed with the mother or by authority of the court
- A *guardian* as appointed through a will or court order
- Certain persons appointed through a care or residence order, e.g. a representative of the local authority.

Note that the Act allows anyone with parental responsibility to act alone, meaning that the consent of only one parent of a legitimate child is necessary. They may also authorize a third party to act on their behalf although they may not surrender responsibility. The Act also allows anyone who has the care of a child to make decisions in the 'best interests' of the child so, for example, a teacher can give consent to a life-saving or life-preserving procedure.

Children in need

The Act defines 'children in need' as being those who are:

- unlikely to achieve or maintain a reasonable standard of health or development or it will be impaired without the provision of services by a local authority
- disabled.

The Act requires local authorities to:

- identify such children and keep a voluntary register of all disabled children
- make assessments of need
- provide appropriate services
- promote care within the family
- publicize services available
- ensure that families receive all relevant information.

Note that despite this increase in responsibilities for local authorities, there was no corresponding increase in resources.

The Act also brought in three new protection orders (Table 14.2) and it should be noted that the checklist discussed earlier does not apply to emergency proceedings.

Finally, the Act also covers other areas such as foster homes, childminding and day care.

TABLE 14.2 Protection orders (PO)

	Emergency PO (EPO)	Police PO (PPO)	Child Assessment Order (CAO)
Duration	8 days – renewable for further 7 days	72 hours – not renewable	7 days – not renewable
Applicant	Anyone who then gains 'parental responsibility' – usually the local authority	Police officer	Local authority or NSPCC
Apply to	Magistrates' Court	None – police officer makes decision	Magistrates' Court
Purpose	Prevent significant harm and/or allow investigation, including medical and psychiatric examination Replaced the 'place of safety' order	As EPO	Non-urgent medical, social or other investigation

NSPCC, National Society for the Prevention of Cruelty to Children

CHILDREN (SCOTLAND) ACT 1995

The *Children (Scotland) Act 1995* has many provisions similar to those in the *Children Act 1989*. However, child protection procedures in Scotland are very different in that the system revolves around the Reporter to the Children's Panel.

THE REPORTER

This is a nationally appointed post and he considers reports from anyone with an interest in the welfare of a particular child. This includes teachers, social workers and the police. The Reporter must decide whether:

1. there are grounds for referral to a children's hearing – these include the commission of a criminal offence, lack of parental control and misuse of drugs or alcohol
2. there is a need for compulsory

measures of supervision – either in the home, with foster carers or in a children's home. 'Supervision' includes medical treatment, protection and control of a child.

If there are no grounds, then the Reporter either takes no action or refers the case to the local authority.

CHILDREN'S HEARINGS

These are held in private and parents can accompany the child, unless they are involved in the proceeding such as NAI where the alleged perpetrator is the parent. There is no legal representation. The panel consists of three trained and lay people of mixed sex and varied background. The Reporter gives the grounds for referral and a decision is made whether or not a compulsory supervision order is necessary. If the grounds are disputed, then the case is referred to the Sheriff.

PROOF HEARINGS

At these hearings, the Reporter represents the child and legal representation is allowed. The standard of proof required is the civil standard, i.e. 'balance of probabilities' (see Ch. 2), and dress is informal, although evidence is given on oath. The Sheriff then decides if the grounds are adequate. If they are, the case returns to the children's hearing; if not, then the referral is discharged.

PLACE OF SAFETY

The *Children (Scotland) Act* gives the police the power to remove children in need of emergency care to a place of safety, which can be either a police station or a hospital. Social workers can also remove children but they must first appear before a Justice to get authorization and it is only granted where it has not been possible or practicable to get a child protection order from a Sheriff. This is the same as the EPO in English and Welsh law and transfers parental responsibility to the applicant.

CHILD PROTECTION REGISTER

The Child Protection Register is also known as the 'At Risk' register and has the following functions:

- To provide a list of all children who have either been subjected to, or are thought to be at risk of, abuse
- To provide statistical data
- To assist in making the diagnosis of child abuse although it is important to note that it has limited value in this respect.

If a child is not on the register, it does not mean that he is not being abused, it may simply mean that it has not yet been brought to the attention of the relevant authorities. However, the reverse may also be true – inclusion on the register does not automatically mean that he is being abused but it should raise suspicion.

The register is maintained by the social services and it must be available 24 hours a day to relevant parties (e.g. Accident & Emergency departments).

MAKING THE DIAGNOSIS

- Take a full history, making a note of any risk factors.
- Remember that physical abuse is often associated with other forms

of abuse and that it can both recur and escalate. The aim is recognition and early intervention. This is particularly important in infants and toddlers who are at a greater risk of serious injury or death than older children.

- Fully undress and carefully examine the whole child if you have *any* suspicions.
- Plot the growth on a centile chart.
- Make legible, dated, contemporaneous, detailed notes with drawings of any injuries, showing measurements.
- Check the 'At Risk' register.
- Check for coagulation defects.
- Perform a skeletal survey if you have *any* suspicions.
- Get the paediatric teams and child protection agencies involved *early*.

THE CHILDREN ACTS IN PRACTICE

If you assess a child and believe him to be at 'significant risk' of harm, then your options are as outlined in Figure 14.6.

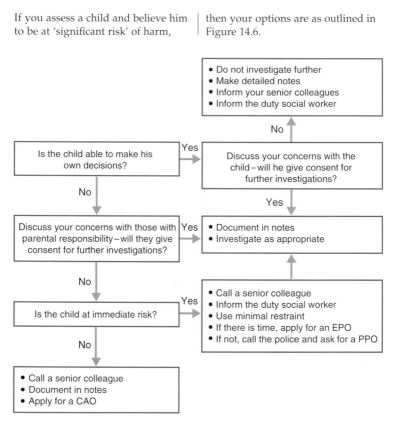

Fig. 14.6 Assessment of a child considered to be at 'significant risk' of harm. CAO, child assessment order; EPO, emergency protection order; PPO, police protection order

Reference

1. Williams RA. Injuries in infants
   and small children resulting
   from witnessed and corroborated
   free falls. J Trauma 1991;
   31: 1350–1356

Further reading

Department of Health. Children Act
  1989 – guidance and regulations.
  London: HMSO, 1991
McLay WDS. Clinical forensic
  medicine, 2nd edn. London:
  Greenwich Medical Media, 1996

CHAPTER 15

THE MENTAL HEALTH ACTS

INTRODUCTION

Of all the chapters in this book, this is the one most certain to be updated as the *Mental Health Act 1983* is currently under review and will be reformed in the near future. However, this Act and its Scottish equivalent, the *Mental Health Act 1984 (Scotland)*, are such important pieces of legislation that any book covering the legal aspects of medicine would be incomplete if it did not discuss them. This chapter also includes an outline of the proposed reforms. Note that the Acts apply equally to children as to adults, with the usual provisos regarding competence (see Ch. 5). Note also that the majority of patients who suffer from a mental disorder are treated and admitted to hospital informally and with their consent, without recourse to these Acts.

THE MENTAL HEALTH ACT (MHA) 1983

The *MHA 1983* replaced the *MHA 1959*, which in turn replaced the *Lunacy Act 1890*. It has 149 sections and is divided into 10 parts:

- **Part I:** (Section 1): Defines mental disorder
- **Part II:** (Sections 2–34): Compulsory admission to hospital and guardianship
- **Part III:** (Sections 35–55): Remand to hospital through criminal proceedings
- **Part IV:** (Sections 56–64): Consent to treatment
- **Part V:** (Sections 65–79): Mental health review tribunals
- **Part VI:** (Sections 80–92): Movement of patients around and in and out of England and Wales
- **Part VII:** (Sections 93–113): The Court of Protection, which is an office of the Supreme Court (see Ch. 1) that manages the property and affairs of detained persons. It has wide-ranging powers, including the buying and selling of property and investments
- **Part VIII:** (Sections 114–125): Duties of the local authorities and the Secretary of State
- **Part IX:** (Sections 126–130): Criminal offences such as forgery and ill treatment of patients
- **Part X:** (Sections 131–149): Miscellaneous matters such as the management of mentally ill patients in public places and the statutory protection of healthcare professionals from litigation for acts done in pursuance of the Act.

THE MHA AND CLINICAL PRACTICE

SECTION 1 – DEFINITION OF MENTAL DISORDER

This section is particularly important as a person must be suffering from a mental disorder as defined by the Act before compulsory admission to hospital or guardianship can be considered:

- *Mental disorder* means mental illness, arrested or incomplete development of mind, psychopathic disorder or any other disorder or disability of mind.
- *Severe mental impairment* means a state of arrested or incomplete development of mind which includes severe impairment of intelligence and social functioning and is associated with abnormally aggressive or seriously irresponsible conduct on the part of the person concerned.
- *Mental impairment* means a state of arrested or incomplete development of mind which includes significant impairment of intelligence and social functioning and is associated with abnormally aggressive or seriously irresponsible conduct on the part of the person concerned.
- *Psychopathic disorder* means a persistent disorder or disability of mind (whether or not including significant impairment of intelligence) that results in abnormally aggressive or seriously irresponsible conduct on the part of the person concerned.

Note

The Act also states that 'A person may not be regarded as suffering from mental disorder by reason of promiscuity or other immoral conduct, sexual deviancy or dependence on alcohol or drugs'.

SECTION 2 – ADMISSION FOR ASSESSMENT

- *Duration:* Admission for assessment +/– medical treatment for ≤ 28 days
- *Application:* Nearest relative (as defined in s.26) or a social worker approved under s.114 of the Act (Approved Social Worker or ASW)
- *Recommendations:* Two doctors, one of whom must be 'approved' under s.12 of the Act and the other with previous acquaintance of the patient
- *Grounds:* That the patient:
  — is suffering from mental disorder of a nature or degree that warrants detention in hospital for assessment (and treatment) for at least a limited period, and
  — ought to be so detained in the interests of his own health or safety or with a view to the protection of others
- *Right of appeal:* Within 14 days of admission
- *Discharge:* Nearest relative, managers or doctor but the doctor can bar discharge by the nearest relative. The patient must be discharged after 28 days unless he has been further detained under s.3.

Note that if the patient is not sectioned or admitted informally following assessment, then under the Code of Practice, the ASW and doctors must make arrangements for his further care. This is the most commonly used section.

SECTION 3 – ADMISSION FOR TREATMENT

- *Duration:* Admission for treatment *of a mental disorder* for ≤ 6 months unless the section is renewed under s.20(4)
- *Application:* Nearest relative or an ASW
- *Recommendations:* Two doctors, one of whom must be s.12 'approved'
- *Grounds:* That the patient:
  - — is suffering from mental disorder of a nature or degree that makes it appropriate for him to receive treatment, and
  - — in the case of psychopathic disorder or mental impairment, such treatment is likely to alleviate or prevent deterioration of his condition, and
  - — ought to be so detained and treated in the interests of his own health or safety or with a view to the protection of others
- *Right of appeal:* Within the first 6 months and once during each subsequent period for which detention is renewed
- *Discharge:* Nearest relative, managers or doctor but the doctor can bar discharge by the nearest relative.

This is used for patients where the diagnosis is already known.

SECTION 4 – APPLICATION FOR ASSESSMENT IN CASES OF EMERGENCY

- *Duration:* Admission for assessment only for 72 hours
- *Application:* Nearest relative or an ASW
- *Recommendations:* One doctor who is preferably acquainted with the patient. Note that unless a psychiatrist is involved, no bed will be made available so it has limited use and should never be used simply for administrative convenience
- *Grounds:*
  - — as for s.2, and
  - — it is of urgent necessity to admit the patient and that admission under s.2 would involve undesirable delay
- *Discharge:* Automatic after 72 hours unless a second medical recommendation is given and received by the managers within that period.

Note that neither this nor the following sections allow for treatment without consent, but appropriate emergency treatment to contain the patient (e.g. sedation) may be given under common law in the best interests of the patient.

SECTION 5(2) – APPLICATION IN RESPECT OF AN INPATIENT

- *Duration:* Detention of a patient already receiving *any form of inpatient treatment* for ≤ 72 hours, including any period during which a nurse's holding power was used. It cannot be used for outpatients or those attending the Accident & Emergency department

- *Application:* The doctor in charge of the patient, or his nominated deputy, must report to the managers on Form 12 that it appears that the patient presents a danger to himself or others and requires compulsory detention
- *Right of appeal:* None
- *Discharge:* Automatic after 72 hours unless further powers have been taken under s.2 or s.3.

SECTION 5(4) – NURSES HOLDING POWER

This is applicable only to patients already receiving treatment for mental disorder in hospital and it allows a Registered Mental Nurse (including those registered for mental handicap) to detain a patient for ≤ 6 hours from the time that the decision is recorded on Form 13 until a doctor is found. The nurse himself must make the decision and he cannot be instructed to invoke the section by anyone else. It must appear to the nurse:

1. that the patient is suffering from mental disorder to such a degree that it is necessary to immediately restrain him in the interests of his own health or safety or with a view to the protection of others, and
2. that it is not practicable to secure the immediate attendance of a doctor.

Note that the section is an emergency measure that lapses on

the arrival of a doctor. The nurse must then complete Form 16.

SECTION 7 – APPLICATION FOR GUARDIANSHIP

- *Duration:* Allows a patient of ≤ 16 years to be placed under the supervision of a guardian for 6 months unless it is renewed
- *Application:* Nearest relative or an ASW
- *Recommendations:* Two doctors, one of whom must be s.12 'approved' and they must have seen the patient together or within 5 days of one another
- *Grounds:* That the patient is suffering from a mental disorder and that it is necessary for him to have a guardian
- *Right of appeal:* Once in each 6 month period
- *Discharge:* Nearest relative, authority or doctor
- *Powers of guardians:* Defined in s.8 – to require the patient to:
  — reside at a specified place
  — attend specified places at specified times, e.g. hospital or school
  — allow access to any doctor, ASW or other specified person.

A summary of the main sections of the Act applicable in clinical practice is provided in Table 15.1.

SECTION 12 – MEDICAL RECOMMENDATIONS

This grants approval for the purposes of the Act to suitable doctors from the Secretary of State. It recognizes

TABLE 15.1 Summary of main sections of the Act applicable in clinical practice

	Section 2	Section 3	Section 4	Section 5(2)	Section 5(4)	Section 7
Type of application	Admission for assessment and treatment	Admission for treatment	Emergency admission for assessment	Detention of an inpatient	Nurses holding power	Guardianship
Application	Nearest relative or an ASW	Nearest relative or an ASW	Nearest relative or an ASW	Report from doctor in charge of patient	None	Nearest relative or an ASW
Medical recommendations required	2, of which ≥1 must be s.12 approved	2, of which ≥1 must be s.12 approved	1, who should preferably know the patient	1	None	2, of which ≥1 must be s.12 approved
Length of detention	≤28 days	≤6 months	≤72 hours	≤72 hours	≤6 hours	≤6 months
Renewable?	Must convert to s.3	Yes	Must convert to s.2 or s.3	Must convert to s.2 or s.3	Must convert to s.5(2)	Yes
Application to tribunal?	Within 14 days	Once in each 6 month period	No	No	No	Once in each 6 month period

that the doctor has special experience in the diagnosis and treatment of mental disorder. Where two doctors are required, they should not normally be associated but two doctors from the same hospital can give the recommendations in cases of emergency.

SECTION 139

This prohibits proceedings against healthcare professionals for any action related to the Act, unless it was done in bad faith or without due care. It means that civil actions may only be brought with the permission of the High Court and criminal proceedings must have the consent of the Director of Public Prosecutions. However, it is important to note that failure to apply the Act may also give rise to litigation.

THE MHA AND FORENSIC PRACTICE

The following sections apply to people who are believed to be suffering from a mental disorder and who have been accused or found guilty of a criminal offence.

SECTION 35 – REMAND TO HOSPITAL FOR A REPORT

- *Purpose:* Allows a Magistrates' or Crown Court to remand an accused person who is either awaiting sentence or trial for an imprisonable offence, to a specified hospital for a report within 7 days
- *Recommendation:* Either written or oral evidence from one doctor that the patient is suffering from a mental disorder and that it would not be practical to obtain a report on bail
- *Duration:* Lasts 28 days and is renewable at 28-day intervals for ≤ 12 weeks by application to court although the court can end the remand at any time.

If it becomes clear after the assessment that the prisoner requires treatment, then it may be given if he gives consent. If he refuses treatment, then the case must be returned to court in order to obtain a treatment order under s.36, although the prisoner himself does not need to appear.

Note that if the order came from a Magistrates' Court and the case is subsequently committed to the Crown Court, then the order cannot be extended as the Magistrates' Court then loses jurisdiction. Theoretically, this means that the patient must then be either returned to custody or given bail, either of which may be very inappropriate for a mentally disordered patient. In practice, the patient is usually remanded to custody then immediately returned under s.48.

SECTION 36 – REMAND TO HOSPITAL FOR TREATMENT

- *Purpose:* Allows a Crown Court only to remand an accused person who is awaiting trial for any imprisonable offence except murder, to hospital for treatment within 7 days.

(Note that this means that for cases still at the Magistrates' Court or where the charge is murder, there is no treatment order available preconviction unless the prisoner is then detained under s.3. The legitimacy of this practice has been disputed although it has yet to be tested in court.)

- *Reports:* Two reports, at least one of which must come from a s. 12 approved doctor
- *Duration:* Lasts 28 days and is renewable at 28-day intervals for ≤ 12 weeks by application to court but the court can terminate the remand at any time.

SECTION 37 – HOSPITAL AND GUARDIANSHIP ORDERS

- *Purpose:* Allows a court to order hospital admission or reception into guardianship as an alternative to a prison sentence for prisoners found guilty of any imprisonable offence except murder. The prisoner must be admitted within 28 days
- *Grounds:* As for s.3
- *Reports:* As for s.36
- *Duration:* ≤ 6 months – renewable for a further 6 months then annually

- *Right of appeal:* Not until the second 6-month period but it ceases to have effect if the prisoner appeals successfully against conviction.

Under s.41, the Crown Court may add the restriction that the patient may not leave or be transferred without the permission of the Home Secretary based on the oral evidence of one doctor that the patient presents a serious threat to public safety.

SECTIONS 47 AND 48 – TRANSFER OF PRISONERS TO HOSPITAL

- *Purpose:* Allows the urgent transfer of prisoners suffering from a mental disorder to hospital on a warrant from the Home Office. Section 47 refers to sentenced prisoners; s.48 to others, including those on remand. It allows compulsory treatment to be given without consent
- *Reports:* Both require two, one of which must be from a s.12 approved doctor
- *Duration:* No time limit
- *Right of appeal:* Within the first 6 months.

The Home Secretary can restrict discharge under s.49, which is applicable up to the expected date of release.

SECTION 135 – REMOVING PATIENTS TO HOSPITAL

If it is suspected that a person who is believed to be suffering from a

mental disorder is being ill-treated, neglected or not properly controlled, or he lives alone and is unable to care for himself, then the ASW should be informed. The ASW can then request a magistrate's warrant to allow a police officer to enter the premises, by force if necessary, and remove that person to a 'place of safety' that for this section is usually the local psychiatric facility. The ASW and a doctor must accompany the officer. The person can be detained ≤72 hours until a mental health assessment can be performed and another section applied (e.g. s.2). Treatment can only be given with consent.

SECTION 136 – PERSONS IN PUBLIC PLACES

This authorizes a police officer to remove a person that he believes to be suffering from a mental disorder from a public place to a 'place of safety' for ≤72 hours for assessment as above. The officer must believe that the person is in immediate need of care and control and/or presents a danger to himself and/or others. For this section, the 'place of safety' refers to a hospital (usually the local psychiatric facility), a police station, certain types of residential accommodation provided by the local authority or any other place deemed suitable by the police, including a private residence if the occupier agrees. Note that the Home Office advises police to take the person to hospital[1] and the Code of Practice recommends that a local policy be agreed between the hospital(s), police and social services regarding the preferred places of safety and individual responsibilities.

For both s.135 and s.136, if the patient leaves, he can be retaken by the person last in charge of his custody, a police officer or the ASW.

THE MHA AND CONSENT

Detention under the MHA does not necessarily mean that a patient is incapable of giving informed consent, but the Act provides that treatment can be given where the patient is either incompetent (see Ch. 5) or refuses to give consent. Under Section 63, 'the consent of the patient shall not be required for any medical treatment given to him for the mental disorder from which he is suffering'. A detained person can be treated even if he refuses such treatment and he may be restrained if necessary. However, any such treatment must be reasonable, i.e. in accordance with accepted medical practice (see Ch. 9) and the restraint should be sufficient only to allow the proposed procedure to be carried out. Although s.63 refers to mental disorders only, it has been used to treat physical disorders where they are believed to either contribute towards, or be symptomatic of, the mental problem. This has included the force-feeding of anorexics but it cannot be used where the physical problem is unconnected. In the case of *Re C* in 1993,[2] a schizophrenic with gangrene in his foot refused to consent to an amputation and sought injunction to prevent it being done without his express consent. The judge ruled that he could refuse consent despite suffering from

delusions, as he was capable of understanding what was proposed and the consequences of his refusal.

> **Note**
>
> The MHA only applies to the treatment of mental disorder, NOT physical.

Note that a patient who is not capable of giving consent to his admission through reason of his mental disorder may still be admitted informally if he is admitted to an unlocked ward and does not attempt to leave or refuse treatment given in his 'best interests'. If such a patient does attempt to leave and he is considered to be a danger to himself or others, he can then be detained under s.5 of the MHA.

The following sections refer to specified treatments and are applicable only to patients detained under s.3 or s.37.

SECTION 57 – TREATMENT REQUIRING CONSENT AND A SECOND OPINION

This applies to all patients undergoing:

- any surgical operation for destroying brain tissue or its function
- surgical implantation of hormones to reduce male sex drive.

Neither operation can proceed without:

1. informed consent from the patient on a Form 38
2. written certification from one approved, independent doctor and two lay persons (as defined in the Act) that the patient can and has given informed consent
3. certification from the approved doctor on a Form 39 that the treatment is necessary having consulted two other persons involved in the patient's care – one of whom must be a nurse and the other either a nurse or a doctor.

SECTION 58 – TREATMENT REQUIRING CONSENT OR A SECOND OPINION

This applies to specified treatments defined in the Act and Regulations, for example electroconvulsive therapy and the administration of medicine by any means if the patient refuses to take it. Medicine may be given for 3 months without consent but after that time, it may not be given unless:

- the patient has given his informed consent on a Form 38 or
- the approved doctor has certified in writing on a Form 39 after consultation as above, that the patient is incapable of giving informed consent but that the treatment is necessary.

Note that the patient has a statutory right under s.60 to withdraw consent obtained under s.57 or s.58 at any time.

SECTION 62 – URGENT TREATMENT

Treatment which is otherwise restricted by s.57 and s.58 may be given to a detained patient without either formal consent or a second opinion if it is deemed necessary to:

1. save the patient's life
2. prevent a serious deterioration in the patient's condition
3. prevent serious suffering
4. prevent the patient from becoming a hazard to himself or others.

Note that only treatment that is neither 'irreversible' nor 'hazardous' may be given in events 2–4 but the Act does not specify what treatment may or may not be used.

MENTAL HEALTH REVIEW TRIBUNALS

These are independent bodies appointed by the Lord Chancellor. They consist of a psychiatrist and a lay member, and are presided over by a barrister or, for s.41 cases, a judge. They provide a right of appeal against detention or guardianship and the patient can apply for legal aid and be legally represented at the tribunal. Either the patient or the nearest relative can make applications; hospital managers or the Secretary of State may also refer patients.

THE MHA COMMISSION

This is a special health authority that consists of lawyers, nurses, psychiatrists, psychologists, social workers and lay people. It is responsible to the Secretary of State and its functions are to:

1. appoint independent doctors to give second opinions on points of consent
2. review the treatment of long-term patients
3. visit and interview inmates of psychiatric hospitals and nursing homes
4. investigate complaints made by and about detainees
5. prepare the code of practice.

PROPOSED REFORMS

The proposed changes are aimed at making application of the MHA easier:

- The emphasis will be on the 'best interests' of the patient rather than the protection of others, although hopefully it will address both.
- The definition of mental illness will be much broader and include personality disorders, although it will exclude sexual deviancy and misuse of drugs and alcohol as before.
- There will be a simpler template for 'formal assessment' with the initial assessment in *all* cases lasting for ≤ 7 days followed by a 21-day care and treatment order, issued by an independent reviewer that is applicable in both civil and criminal settings. Thus, there will no longer be a division between clinical and forensic practice.
- An individual care plan of 'direct therapeutic benefit' must be produced and if the mental disorder itself is not treatable, then management must be aimed at 'behaviours arising from the disorder'.
- Care and treatment orders beyond 28 days will only be made by the new Mental Disorder Tribunal or the courts.
- The 'nearest relative' will be replaced by a 'nominated person'.
- There will be a greater focus on care in the community and its legalization.

THE MENTAL HEALTH ACT (MHA) 1984 (SCOTLAND)

This has the same basic principles as the English Act and contains the same definitions of mental disorder. Note that appeals are heard by the Sheriff or the Mental Welfare Commission, rather than a tribunal. The important sections that relate to clinical practice are as follows.

SECTION 18 – ADMISSION FOR TREATMENT

- This is equivalent to the English s.3 and allows admission for treatment for ≤ 6 months.
- The application may be made by the nearest relative or a mental health officer (MHO), who is equivalent to an ASW.
- It is heard in the Sheriff Court (see Ch. 1) and must be accompanied by two medical recommendations, of which one must be from a doctor approved under s.20, which is the equivalent to the English s.12.
- The order can be renewed for a further 6 months, then annually.

SECTION 24 – APPLICATION FOR ASSESSMENT IN CASES OF EMERGENCY

- This allows admission for assessment for 72 hours and is equivalent to the English s.4.
- The application may be made by the nearest relative or an MHO but it only needs to be supported by one doctor who need not be acquainted with the patient.
- The recommendation should be made on Form A.
- The patient must be discharged after 72 hours unless the second medical recommendation is given and received by the managers within that period, converting it to s.26.

SECTION 26 – ADMISSION FOR ASSESSMENT

- This allows admission for assessment +/– medical treatment for ≤ 28 days and is the equivalent of the English s.2.
- The application may be made by the nearest relative or the MHO.
- It must be supported by two doctors, one of whom must be 'approved' under s.20 of the Act.
- Detention of the patient for longer than 28 days requires a s.18 application.

SECTION 117 – REMOVING PATIENTS TO HOSPITAL

This is equivalent to the English s.135.

SECTION 118 – PERSONS IN PUBLIC PLACES

This is equivalent to the English s.136.

WHEN TO APPLY THE MHA

- *Section 2 or 26* (Scotland) should be used where:
  — the diagnosis is not clear
  — this is a first admission
  — a thorough inpatient assessment is required
- *Section 3 or 18* (Scotland) should be used for patients:
  — with a known diagnosis
  — who have been assessed under s.2 or s.26 and have been found to require a further period of detention for treatment. Note that there is no need to wait for the 28 days to expire for applying for s.3 or s.18
- *Section 4 or 24* (Scotland) should be used only in genuine emergencies – not simply because it is difficult to obtain a second medical recommendation.

References

1. Fahy TA. The police as a referral agency for psychiatric emergencies – a review. Med Sci Law 1989; 29(4): 315–322
2. *Re C (Adult: Refusal of treatment)* [1994] 1 All ER 819, (1993) 15 BMLR 77

Further reading

The Code of Practice, Mental Health Act 1983. London: HMSO, 1999

Useful website

Proposed reforms:
www.doh.gov.uk/mentalhealth.htm

CHAPTER 16

THE LAW RELATING TO ALCOHOL AND DRIVING

INTRODUCTION

Alcohol is the most commonly abused substance in the United Kingdom yet, unlike most other drugs, it is freely available. Crime statistics show that alcohol consumption is associated with criminal behaviour, particularly violent assaults, and it is the cause of many serious road accidents. Almost a third of medical and surgical admissions to hospital are for problems related to alcohol, but the healthcare profession has been notoriously poor at detecting and addressing these problems.

METABOLISM OF ALCOHOL

An alcohol is any substance that contains a hydroxyl group attached to a carbon atom and although there is no legal definition, it is usually considered to relate to one specific alcohol – ethanol. Some knowledge of the metabolism of alcohol is important, particularly in relation to the stages of acute and chronic alcoholism and to drink-driving offences.

The blood alcohol level peaks at 30–90 minutes on an empty stomach (Fig. 16.1) but it depends on:

- the rate of absorption as the elimination is very slow
- prior blood alcohol level

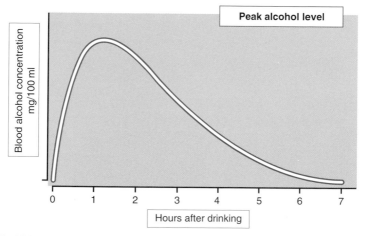

Peak alcohol level

Blood alcohol concentration mg/100 ml

Hours after drinking

Fig. 16.1 Blood alcohol curve

- the duration of alcohol consumption – if the rate of consumption is low then the rates of absorption and elimination are similar and the peak is lower
- the strength of the alcohol – the optimum is 20% as greater concentrations cause mucosal secretion and pyloric spasm and lower concentrations cause dilution, both of which delay absorption
- the type of beverage – beer contains soluble nutrients which delay absorption
- sex – for the same amount of alcohol, the peak level in women is higher as they have a higher fat:water index and alcohol is not distributed in fat
- body weight – the lower the weight, the higher the alcohol concentration as there is less body water to dilute it
- food in the stomach
- physiological factors, e.g. gastric blood supply
- genetic variation, e.g. enzyme levels
- any condition that increases gastric emptying as absorption is greatest in the duodenum, e.g.

previous gastrectomy or drugs such as metoclopramide.

ELIMINATION OF ALCOHOL

The liver detoxifies 95% of the alcohol ingested, with 90% of the remainder being excreted by the kidney. The rest is eliminated in the breath and sweat. The rate of elimination in a normal person varies from 12 to 25 mg/100 ml of blood/hour, with an average of 15, which for a 70 kg man corresponds to one unit per hour. In chronic alcoholics, this rate rises to up to 40 mg/100 ml/hour due to enzyme induction. Elimination is not linear and varies with the absolute level of blood alcohol, but 15 mg/100 ml/hour is usually a good estimate when attempting to back-calculate blood or breath levels.

> ⚠ There are so many variables to take into account when attempting to back-calculate blood alcohol levels that it is *rarely* a useful exercise.

ACUTE EFFECTS OF ALCOHOL

Alcohol is a central nervous system depressant, affecting the highest centres first, and the initial excitatory effects are caused by depression of the inhibitory centres. The effects are dose dependent but there is huge interperson variation. Chronic alcoholics develop tolerance so larger amounts must be consumed to achieve the same effects. The relationship of blood alcohol level and behaviour is shown in Table 16.1.

There is a strong correlation between alcohol consumption and crime. In 1989, the BMA estimated

TABLE 16.1 Blood alcohol level and behaviour	
mg/100 ml	Effects
< 50	Not obvious, talkative, driving skills deteriorate
50–100	'Dizzy and delightful' – slurred speech, bravado; some loss of coordination
100–150	'Drunk and disorderly' – marked loss of coordination, staggering gait, disorientation
150–200	Nausea; non-cooperative; loss of inhibition
200–300	'Dead drunk' – probable coma; vomiting, stupor; incontinence
300–400	Coma; impaired respiration; loss of reflexes
> 400	'Devil's disciple' – dead

that alcohol was involved in 60–70% of murders, 75% of stabbings and 50% of fights or domestic violence.[1]

CHRONIC EFFECTS OF ALCOHOL

There is a complex relationship between alcohol consumption and various diseases but both the amount and frequency of alcohol consumption are important factors in the size and direction of the effect. Any research is complicated by the following:

- Except for violent deaths attributable to acute intoxication, the risks and benefits of alcohol consumption are likely to change with time.
- Quantitative assessment of drinking is generally based on self-reporting, which may lead to some misclassification.
- Alcohol consumption is usually associated with other lifestyle factors such as smoking or profession.
- Other constituents of alcoholic beverages may also affect the risks of disease.
- Drinking habits may change with age.

For overall mortality, the curve is U-shaped, with an increase in all causes of mortality at higher levels of consumption. However, drinkers of small to moderate amounts of alcohol tend to have lower total mortality than non-drinkers, probably due to a fall in the risk of coronary heart disease. This cardioprotective effect seems to be mediated through an increase in the level of high density lipoprotein (HDL) cholesterol although there may also be other antiatherogenic and antithrombotic mechanisms. It is independent of sex and the type of alcoholic beverage. It is not known whether alcohol also reduces the relative risk of coronary heart disease in younger people as most studies have been done in people over 40. Even if it does, other causes of alcohol-related death, especially accidents, are likely to outweigh any possible benefit, given that the risk of cardiac-related death is lower anyway.

Some diseases are almost exclusively related to alcohol consumption, such as cirrhosis and Wernicke's encephalopathy, and alcohol has been shown to be a risk factor for various types of cancer, including cancer of the mouth, oesophagus, pharynx, larynx, liver and breast cancer in women. Until 1984, chronic alcoholism could be given as a cause of death but it must now be reported to the Coroner (see Ch. 11).

Hazards associated with alcoholism

- Car accidents – either as a pedestrian or driver
- Falls
- Burns
- Hypothermia
- Susceptibility to infections
- Liver, stomach and brain damage
- Withdrawal fits

The current recommendations for maximum alcohol consumption are 21 units (168 g of ethanol) a week for men and 14 units (112 g ethanol) a week for women. However, setting a limit of 3 units a

TABLE 16.2 Alcohol content of some beverages

Beverage	Alcohol content
Beer, lager and cider*	2.5–4.5% v/v
Table wine	8–12% v/v
Fortified wines	20% v/v
Spirits	37–40% v/v
Liqueurs (and rum)	45% v/v or more

*Beware 'super-strength' which are *much* higher

day for men and 2 units a day for women might be more prudent to avoid 'binge drinking'.

Alcohol misuse is common – in 1995, 4% of adults were dependent[1] but it is probably vastly underreported as healthcare professionals may not ask about alcohol intake and even if they do, the patient may not give a true approximate. This is compounded by the fact that many healthcare professionals are unaware of the unit values for common alcoholic drinks (Table 16.2). Most wine is 12% alcohol and a glass is 125 ml (six glasses to a bottle). An average glass of wine therefore contains 15 ml of alcohol, or $1^1/_2$ units. One can of extra strong lager contains 4 units of alcohol.

Note

Alcohol is less dense than water so volume per volume (v/v) alcohol content is not the same as weight per volume (w/v), e.g. 40% v/v whisky actually contains 32 mg of alcohol per 100 ml.

ALCOHOL AND THE HEALTHCARE PROFESSIONAL

In 1997, British Health Authorities were asked to consider the practicality of introducing compulsory liver function tests for all doctors every 2 years to pick up early warning signs of alcohol problems. This followed a fatal accident inquiry into the perioperative deaths of two patients where the surgeon subsequently admitted to having a serious drink problem. It was not instituted, partly because it was felt that it might still fail to identify the minority of those who are alcohol dependent as liver function tests are not specific and may be normalized by a period of abstention.

Alcohol dependence is undoubtedly a problem amongst healthcare professionals and both the General Medical Council (GMC) and the Nursing and Midwifery Council (NMC) advise that healthcare professionals have an ethical obligation to disclose information about a colleague who is putting patients at risk. This also applies to patients who are misusing alcohol yet continue to drive or work in occupations that may put themselves or others at risk. The advice from the GMC and the Driving and Vehicle Licensing Agency (DVLA) is clear but healthcare professionals often seem reluctant to follow it.

If the patient works in a hazardous occupation, then you have a duty to inform his employer, preferably via the occupational health department. This is 'disclosure in the public interest' (see Ch. 6) but you must warn the patient that you intend to do so and confirm it in writing. The same advice applies if a patient is acutely intoxicated and you have reason to believe that he intends to drive. You have an ethical duty to inform the police but again you must warn the patient that you intend to do so.

DRINK AND DRIVING

Over 1000 people are killed in the United Kingdom each year as a result of drinking and driving and it causes 10% of all road accidents resulting in injury. At the legal limit, the chances of a serious accident are twice normal but at twice the legal limit, the risk is 20 times greater. Alcohol impairs vision, lengthens reaction time, reduces coordination and makes drivers think that they are invincible – a lethal combination. Driving while under the influence of drugs is also an offence and although the scale of the problem is not known, it is likely that it is very high. Drivers who drink or who are under the influence of drugs can be prosecuted under the *Road Traffic Act* of 1988.

ROAD TRAFFIC ACT OF 1988

Section 7(6): A person who without reasonable excuse fails to provide a specimen when required to do so in pursuance of this Section is guilty of an offence.

SECTION 4 OFFENCES

It is an offence under Section 4 of the Road Traffic Act 1988 to drive a motor vehicle whilst impaired through alcohol or drugs.

There are three pieces of evidence required to prove impairment under Section 4 (evidence from the arresting officer, evidence from the doctor and toxological evidence), although a prosecution can proceed with only two.

Evidence from the arresting officer

This is particularly important for drugs such as cannabis, which may have only a short period of intoxication.

Evidence from the doctor

Impairment *must* be assessed by a 'medically qualified person' because it may be the result of an underlying physical or mental illness or injury (see box).

The doctor must get informed consent (see Ch. 5), ensuring that the person is fully aware of the possible consequences, and write it in the notes. He must also tell the person that anything said during the assessment

Conditions that may result in impairment

- Drug intoxication – both prescribed (e.g. benzodiazepines or antihistamines) and illicit (e.g. cannabis)
- Drug and alcohol withdrawal
- Metabolic disorders, e.g. hypo- or hyperglycaemia, uraemia, porphyria, Addison's disease, thyrotoxicosis, hepatic failure
- Head injury
- Neurological disorders, e.g. Parkinson's disease, multiple sclerosis, epilepsy, vertigo, transient ischaemic attack
- High fever
- Cardiac disease, e.g. dysrhythmias
- Fatigue
- Carbon monoxide poisoning
- Mental illness, e.g. schizophrenia, hypomania

cannot be regarded as confidential and that he can request his own doctor to perform the assessment if this will not delay the procedure. The examination must be meticulously performed and documented, as it is very likely that the doctor will have to defend his opinions in court. The actual examination is beyond the scope of this book but can be found in the books in the Further reading list.

Toxicological evidence

At the end of the examination, the doctor must advise the custody sergeant whether there is evidence that alcohol or drugs have been taken recently and, if so, whether or not the ability of the person to drive was impaired. If there is evidence, then the sergeant will continue with the blood/urine option as in Section 5.

SECTION 5 OFFENCES

> It is an offence under Section 5 of the Road Traffic Act 1988 to drive a motor vehicle with more than the legal limits of alcohol (see Table 16.3).

In 1996, the British Medical Association (BMA) called for the limit to be lowered to 50 mg/100 ml following evidence that any detectable blood alcohol increases the risk of drivers being involved in accidents. It has yet to be changed and whether lowering the limit would substantially affect the more serious offenders is difficult to judge. Those who believe that their skills are unimpaired by their current levels of drinking would not reduce their intake unless they thought that there was a high risk of getting caught, so a lower limit might have to operate alongside random breath testing in order to be effective. This is not yet permissible in the United Kingdom despite being common practice abroad, but a person stopped for any reason

may be tested at the discretion of the police officer. The roadside test is a screening procedure and if it proves negative, the person is allowed to proceed unless there are grounds for suspecting impairment due to drugs. If the driver refuses to perform the roadside test, then he will be arrested on the grounds of 'failure to provide' and taken to the police station. The roadside meter is set at 35 mcg/100 ml breath and gives a green signal if the alcohol content of the breath is well below and yellow if it is near the threshold. If it shows a red signal, the driver will be arrested and taken to the police station for an evidential breath test.

Evidential breath samples are taken by a specially trained police officer (usually the custody sergeant) using an Intoximeter. The accused must give two breath samples and the lower reading is the one accepted. Although the legal limit is 35 mcg/100 ml, no action is taken unless the reading is 40 or over. If the two samples fall between 40 and 50 mcg/100 ml, then the accused is given the option of providing a blood or urine sample or being charged on the basis of the breath sample. If the samples differ by more than a set limit, then the sergeant can require a blood or urine sample, with the type of sample being at his discretion. If the accused does not give a breath sample without reasonable excuse (see box), then he will be charged with 'failure to provide'.

If the accused is in hospital following an accident, then the evidential sample must be of blood and the Accident & Emergency staff

TABLE 16.3 Legal limits of alcohol	
Sample	Legal limit
Breath	35 mcg/100 ml breath
Blood	80 mg/100 ml blood
Urine	107 mg/100 ml urine
Note different units for breath	

Medical reasons for failure to provide a breath sample

- Asthma and other chronic lung problems
- Acute chest infection
- Injury to mouth, lip or face
- Tracheotomy, rib or chest injury
- Neurological problems, e.g. facial palsy
- Obesity
- Small stature
- Angina
- Neck problems, e.g. cervical spondylosis
- Comatose
- Inability to understand warning, e.g. mental disability
- Panic attacks and hyperventilation
- Alcohol intoxication (although this is *not* a 'reasonable excuse')

Note

There is no legal obligation for a doctor to take a blood sample, but there may be moral duty. Where possible, leave it to the FME!

blood sample. If the doctor objects, then the requirement cannot be made. The objection must be on the basis that it would be 'prejudicial to the proper care and treatment of the patient' either to provide the sample or to be given the obligatory warning that he will be prosecuted for 'failure to provide'.

Note

Blood taken for diagnostic purposes cannot be subjected to analysis under the Road Traffic Act.

may be asked to take it. If the accused is able to give informed consent (see Chapter 6), then the doctor must get *specific consent and write it in the notes, ensuring that the patient is fully aware of the possible legal consequences. He must be very clear that this is **not** a therapeutic procedure!* Note that poor comprehension due to intoxication is not a valid excuse. A nurse *must not* take the blood, as the Road Traffic Act states that a 'medically-qualified person' must take the sample. Any swabs used *must* be alcohol-free. If the patient is unconscious, a recent change in the law now allows the doctor to take an evidential sample of blood without consent.

The police are obliged to notify the attending doctor before requiring the patient to provide a

Whether in hospital or in custody, the doctor decides the site of venepuncture and is allowed three attempts to take one sample, which is then divided into two equal parts and labelled. The accused has the option to have one part tested at an independent laboratory from an approved list at his own expense.

Reasons for failure to provide a blood sample

- Needle phobia – this must be genuine and supported either by a psychiatrist's letter or signs of real anxiety and avoidance strategies
- Poor venous access
- Bleeding diatheses

If the accused refuses to give blood without the grounds shown in the box, then he is charged with 'failure to provide'.

If the accused cannot provide a blood sample, the police can request a urine sample. Urine samples are collected by the police officer. The accused is asked to empty his bladder, then the urine that he produces is collected over the next hour *under the supervision* of the police officer. The process is degrading and open to contamination, so is avoided wherever possible. If the accused cannot or will not provide a urine

sample, then he is charged with 'failure to provide', unless there is a medical reason as shown below:

Reasons for failure to provide a urine sample

- Drugs causing urinary retention
- Dehydration
- Neurological problems affecting the bladder
- Catheters
- Embarrassment at providing a sample in front of a member of the opposite sex
- Alcohol intoxication

MEDICAL ASPECTS OF fiTNESS TO DRIVE

Each time a healthcare professional writes a prescription, he should also consider the fact that many different drugs can affect fitness to drive and advise the patient accordingly.

Drugs affecting ability to drive

- Prescribed, e.g. tranquillizers; antiepileptics; antidepressants; antipsychotics; antihistamines; analgesics; anaesthetics
- Illicit, e.g. opiates; cannabis, LSD

Licensing requirements depend on the type of vehicle driven but an ordinary license is valid up to the age of 70 then it must be renewed every 3 years, but this is automatic unless the driver reports a problem. Every license states that a driver is obliged to inform the DVLA of any potential or actual medical disability

that may affect his driving but few are aware of this. If the patient refuses to inform the DVLA and the doctor has concerns, he should proceed as follows:

1. Inform the patient that he has a legal duty to inform the DVLA.
2. If the patient refuses to accept the diagnosis or the associated risks, suggest a second opinion and advise him not to drive until it is obtained.
3. If the patient continues to drive, then try to persuade him not to do so, possibly by involving the next of kin.
4. If the patient still drives, then tell him that the DVLA will be informed.
5. Discuss the matter with his defence organization.
6. Give the medical information to the Medical Adviser at the DVLA.

7. Write to the patient, informing him that he has done so.

In the United Kingdom, the DVLA provides guidelines for doctors entitled *At a Glance Guide to the* *Current Medical Standards of Fitness to Drive.* Some of the medical conditions affecting driving with an ordinary license are shown in Table 16.4.

TABLE 16.4 Medical conditions affecting driving

Disease		Driving restrictions
Epilepsy		Fit-free for ≥ 1 year
Narcolepsy		Yearly medical review once controlled
Chronic neurological disease e.g. Parkinson's; multiple sclerosis		None if medical assessment confirms no impairment
CVA, TIA		Stop ≥ 4/52 then start if no residual disability
Vertigo, Menière's		Stop until symptoms controlled
Benign brain tumours		Stop for 1 year then 3-yearly review
Serious head injury		Stop 6/12 – 1 year
Angina		Stop if rest pain or on driving
Myocardial infarction/CABG		Stop ≥ 4/52
Arrhythmias		Stop until controlled for ≥ 4/52
Syncope		Stop until cause identified and controlled
Hypertension		None unless drugs cause problems
Heart valve disease/HOCM		None
Heart/lung transplant		None
Diabetes	Insulin dependent	Cannot drive light goods or small passenger-carrying vehicles
	Non-insulin dependent	None
Vision	Acuity	At least 6/12
	Fields	At least 120° on the horizontal meridian with no significant field defect within 20° of fixation
	Colour blindness	None
Deafness		None
Mental illness	Psychosis	Stop until medical assessment
	Depression	None unless suicidal
	Schizophrenia	None if controlled
Dementia		Stop until medical assessment
Drugs	Opiates	Stop for 1 year screening
	Cannabis	Stop for 6/12 then screening

CABG, coronary artery bypass graft; CVA, cerebrovascular accident; HOCM, hypertrophic obstructive cardiomyopathy; TIA, transient ischaemic attack

References
1. British Medical Association. Alcohol and accidents. London: BMA, 1989
2. Chick J. Alcohol and driving. In: Medical Commission on the Prevention of Accidents. Medical aspects of fitness to drive. London: HMSO, 1995: pp 157–167

Further reading
Driver and Vehicle Licensing Agency. For medical practitioners: At a glance guide to the current medical standards of fitness to drive. Swansea: Drivers Medical Unit, DVLA, 1998
Knight B. Legal aspects of medical practice, 5th edn. London: Churchill Livingstone, 1999
McLay WDS. Clinical forensic medicine, 2nd edn. London: Greenwich Medical Media, 1996

Useful website
www.dvla.org.uk

CHAPTER 17

THE LAW RELATING TO DRUGS

INTRODUCTION

Writing a prescription is potentially one of the healthcare professional's most hazardous tasks. From overprescribing tablets to someone who later uses them to commit suicide to the patient who forges or changes your prescription, the whole process can be fraught with difficulty. Even if your prescription is perfect, you are still supplying a poison, albeit with the best of intentions, to a patient who neither would nor could have it without your intervention. It is therefore vital for every healthcare professional to have a sound knowledge of both the pharmacology and the legislation surrounding drugs. There are already many excellent pharmacology books so this chapter will concentrate on the legal side.

PRESCRIBING

Prescribing was restricted to doctors and dentists until 1992, when the *Medicinal Products: Prescription by Nurses Act* and subsequent amendments to the Pharmaceutical Services regulations allowed NMC-registered health visitors and district nurses to become nurse prescribers. This government plans to expand nurse prescribing and to extend prescribing rights to other healthcare professionals such as paramedics. Guidance on the prescription of different classes of drug can be found in the *British National Formulary*, the *Nurse Prescribers' Formulary* and in *Medicines, Ethics and Practice: A Guide for Pharmacists*.

Prescriptions are usually written for one particular patient but there is a special type of prescription called 'patient group directions'.

A prescription should:

- Clearly identify the patient for whom it is intended
- Be given, where possible, with the patient's informed consent
- Be clearly written, typed or computer-generated and indelible
- Clearly identify the substance by either its generic or brand name and state the preparation, strength, dose, frequency and route of administration, timing, start and finish dates
- Record the weight of the patient where the dose is weight dependent
- Be signed by the prescriber
- *Not* be a substance to which the patient is known to have an adverse or allergic reaction
- Only be given over the telephone if not previously prescribed in *exceptional* circumstances

Previously known as group protocols, they relate to the supply and administration of a named medicine or vaccine in a known clinical situation where the patients may not be identified prior to arrival, for example group vaccinations at school or in a baby clinic. They must be drawn up by a local senior doctor or dentist and a pharmacist and signed by them.

DISPENSING

Any healthcare professional can legally dispense drugs but the patient has a right to expect that it will be done with the same expertise as a qualified pharmacist, so it should only be done under very rigid guidelines, if at all.

ADMINISTRATION

Any healthcare professional who administers a drug must:

- know the therapeutic use, normal dose, side effects, precautions and contraindications of the drug that he is giving
- ensure that it is the correct patient
- ensure it is the correct prescription
- check the dose, route of administration and timing
- check any calculations necessary with a second healthcare professional
- ensure that there are no contraindications, especially allergies and coexisting treatment
- check the expiry date

- clearly, contemporaneously and accurately record the time, dose and route of administration
- clearly, contemporaneously and accurately record if the drug is not given and the reason, e.g. patient refusal
- note and act upon any adverse reactions.

Note

Never prepare intravenous injections in advance or give an injection prepared by another healthcare professional unless they are present.

MANAGEMENT OF ERRORS IN THE ADMINISTRATION OF MEDICINES

Drug errors by nurses are much more tightly controlled than those by doctors. However, the Professional Conduct Committee of the nursing disciplinary body, the NMC (see Ch. 10) takes care to distinguish between errors occurring as a result of erroneous or incompetent practice, with or without concealment, and those resulting from other causes (e.g. high workload). If there was immediate disclosure in the patient's best interest, this is also taken into account.

COMMITTEE ON SAFETY OF MEDICINES (CSM)

This was established under the *Medicines Act 1968* and its role is to assess the data on each potential new drug for safety, quality and efficacy before it can receive its product licence from the Medicines Control Agency (MCA). The CSM also runs the *Yellow Card* scheme, which is the method by which doctors, dentists, coroners and pharmacists can report any adverse drug reactions (ADRs). They are asked to report *any* possible ADRs in 'new' drugs, i.e. those that are marked with an inverted black triangle (▼) in the *British National Formulary* and any *serious* reaction in 'older' established drugs. Yellow Cards are assessed at the MCA to establish whether or not there is a causal relationship between the drug and the ADR and also look for possible risk factors that might increase the chance of the patient developing a reaction, such as age or concurrent disease. The risk of a newly identified ADR is then assessed in the context of the efficacy of the drug, its known side effects, the target population, the condition it is used to treat and other drugs in the same class. The action then taken depends on the gravity of the reaction. Possible outcomes include:

● The new side effect is listed in the product information
● Use of the drug is changed to maximize the benefit and minimize the risk such as changes to the dose or preparation or it may be restricted to more serious conditions
● Special warnings may be issued
● The drug may be withdrawn if the risk of harm is considered to outweigh the benefit.

ADDICTION AND DRUG DEPENDENCE

The total number of addicts in Great Britain is unknown but in the 6 months leading up to March 1998, 30 000 drug misusers reported for treatment with 54% being under 30.[1] The number continues to rise each year with the problem being greatest in London, Liverpool and Glasgow but fewer inject, possibly in response to fears about HIV transmission. The ratio of males to females is 3:1 and 55% use heroin as the main drug of abuse. About 30% of the UK population have used illicit drugs at some time but misuse of prescription drugs (e.g. benzodiazepines) is probably a far greater problem.

DEPENDENCE SYNDROME

This is defined as compulsion to use drugs with an overriding focus on

Commonly misused drugs

- **Benzodiazepines**, e.g. diazepam (Valium), temazepam
- **Opioids**, e.g. diamorphine (heroin), morphine, pethidine, dihydrocodeine (DF118), buprenorphine (Temgesic)
- **Cannabis**, e.g. 'weed', resin cakes, reefers
- **Cocaine and crack**
- **Methylenedioxymetham-phetamine** (MDMA, Ecstasy), e.g. 'e'
- **Amphetamines**
- Lysergide (lysergic acid diethylamide, LSD) and mescaline
- **Volatile substances**, e.g. glue, aerosols, solvents, petrol

drug-seeking behaviour plus one or more of the following:

- Tolerance – the amount of drug needed to give the desired effect rises
- Withdrawal – both physical and psychological symptoms on stopping use
- Use of drug to relieve or avoid withdrawal symptoms.

ADDICTION IN HEALTHCARE PROFESSIONALS

Healthcare professionals are at particular risk of becoming addicted as they do highly stressful jobs and have a unique access to supplies. The very nature of their roles means that their addiction poses a particular risk to the public. While most recovering addicts can continue to work, a healthcare professional may need to be removed from his environment in order to limit his access to the drugs. In addition, healthcare professionals find it more difficult than most to admit to their addiction and to find effective, confidential treatment that will not jeopardize their future careers. A healthcare professional is unlikely to seek help within his own hospital for fear of stigma, yet an extra-contractual referral means that he must be identified under the NHS reforms.

Addicted healthcare professionals are most frequently exposed in a crisis situation such as stealing drugs or being found intoxicated. An internal investigation then follows which is often a protracted and inefficient method of dealing with what is essentially a medical problem. Treatment is often challenging as the healthcare professional may find the role of patient difficult in itself without the associated high expectations of compliance and recovery. However, research has shown that the outcome of comprehensive treatment is good.[2]

Return to work is possible under strict supervision to protect both the healthcare professional and the public. In the United States, testing for drug and alcohol use in the workplace is routinely employed and this has been instituted in Britain for jobs in which safety is critical. A review of the law suggests that employers in such situations are entitled to test for and enforce strict policies on drug and alcohol use, provided that this has been made explicit in the contract, and that a positive test can be the basis of dismissal.

LEGISLATION

MEDICINES ACT 1968

This was passed in response to the thalidomide disaster with the aim of preventing any further such injuries. Thalidomide was a drug used to relieve morning sickness in early pregnancy but it proved to have dreadful teratogenic side effects. The *Medicines Act 1968* provides a legal framework for the manufacture, licensing, prescription, supply, labelling, packaging and administration of 'medicinal products', defined as being made or supplied solely for administration to an animal or a human for a 'medicinal purpose'. A 'medicinal purpose' is defined as: diagnosing, treating or preventing disease; induction of anaesthesia; contraception or any other permanent or temporary effect on physiological function, so covering a huge number of different products. The *Medicines Act* also:

- established the Medicines Control Agency, the Committee on Safety of Medicines and the British Pharmacopoeia
- controls registration of pharmacists and pharmacies
- controls advertising and sales
- classifies medicines into the categories described below.

Categories

- *Prescription-only medicines (POMs)* – these may only be supplied or administered to a patient on the instruction of a doctor, dentist or nurse prescriber
- *Pharmacy-only medicines (P)* – these may only be bought from a registered primary care pharmacy, under the supervision of a pharmacist
- *General sale list medicines (GSLs)* – this is a very limited list subject to various limitations and can be bought from any retail outlet. Includes all veterinary, herbal and aromatherapy products and also paracetamol, aspirin and cold products

UNLICENSED MEDICINES

These have no product licence and no manufacturer liability. If they are given to a patient, then the prescriber carries full liability and they should only be given on a patient-specific prescription.

> **Note**
>
> All controlled drugs must be kept in a locked receptacle and a car is not regarded as such unless they are further locked within a bag or in the boot of the car.

POISONS ACT 1972

This defines a poison as 'any substance that has a harmful effect on a living system'. It covers all *non-medicinal* poisons and divides them into two parts:

- *Part 1* – these can only be sold by a pharmacist, e.g. strychnine, oxalic acid, phenols
- *Part 2* – these can also be sold by a person on the local authority list, e.g. an ironmonger. These include sulphuric acid, paraquat and formaldehyde.

The purchaser must give his name, address and the purpose for which the poison is intended.

MISUSE OF DRUGS ACT 1971

This Act repealed the *Drugs (Prevention of Misuse) Act 1964* and the *Dangerous Drugs Acts* of 1965 and 1967. It prohibits the possession, supply and manufacture of drugs and other products unless this has been legalized under the *Misuse of Drugs Regulations 1985* (see below). Storage of controlled drugs comes under the *Misuse of Drugs (Safe Custody) Regulations 1973*.

The *Misuse of Drugs Act 1971* applies in Northern Ireland, England, Scotland and Wales and has 40 sections and six schedules, although the following are probably of most relevance to the healthcare professional:

- *Section 1* – this established the Advisory Council on the Misuse of Drugs, which is responsible for a national surveillance of which drugs are being misused, what constitutes misuse and whether or not use of a particular drug causes sufficient harmful effects to have a widespread social impact. The Council should then advise Parliament on the steps necessary to control the problem. They also advise on rehabilitation and treatment facilities and public education.
- *Section 2* – this section divides controlled drugs into three categories as shown in Table 17.1. These categories determine the penalties for illegal possession and supply but the Act allows the category of a drug to be changed and for it to be released from control as new evidence appears.
- *Sections 3, 4 and 5* – these control the import and export, supply, destruction, possession and trafficking of controlled drugs.

TABLE 17.1 Categories of controlled drugs

- **Class A**, e.g. heroin, morphine, cocaine, crack, opium, pethidine, LSD, methadone, mescaline, injectable amphetamines
- **Class B**, e.g. oral amphetamines, cannabis, codeine, dihydrocodeine, ecstasy (MDMA)
- **Class C**, e.g. methaqualone, benzodiazepines

Maximum penalty		Possession	Trafficking
Class A:	Summary	6 months/£2000	7 years/seizure of assets
	Indictment	7 years/seizure of assets	Life/seizure of assets
Class B:	Summary	3 months/£500	6 months/£2000
	Indictment	5 years/seizure of assets	14 years/seizure of assets
Class C:	Summary	3 months/£200	2 years/seizure of assets

LSD, lysergic acid diethylamide; MDMA, methylenedioxymethamphetamine

- *Section 6* – this prohibits the cultivation of cannabis plants.
- *Section 7* – this defines the exemptions granted by the Home Office to allow certain people to possess certain controlled drugs.
- The Act also allows the police or 'other authorized person' to enter the premises of anybody producing or supplying drugs and see any relevant documentation, and to search anyone that they have 'reasonable grounds' to suspect may be carrying controlled drugs. This search also extends to their vehicle.
- Under the Act, a doctor can be prevented from prescribing, administering or supplying controlled drugs if that doctor:
  — fails to notify an addict under the *Misuse of Drugs (Notification and Supply to Addicts) Regulations 1973* or treats an addict with heroin or cocaine for anything other than organic disease (s.13)
  — is found guilty of an offence under the Act (s.12)
  — has had his practice limited by the General Medical Council (see Ch. 10), e.g. for irresponsible prescribing.
- *Section 14* – if a doctor is prohibited under the Act, he can appeal to a tribunal of five people, which includes doctors and lawyers. The hearing is private and the doctor can be legally represented. If this procedure fails, then the doctor can appeal to an advisory body whose decision is final.
- *Section 15* – if a doctor's practice is considered to be dangerous and worthy of rapid curtailment, the case can be referred to a professional panel, where again the doctor can be legally represented. The panel can issue a temporary direction, which prohibits the doctor from prescribing or supplying controlled drugs for 6 weeks, although this is subject to 28-day extensions until he appears before the tribunal.

MISUSE OF DRUGS REGULATIONS 1985

These are divided into schedules that allow different classes of people to possess and supply controlled drugs.

- *Schedule 1* – this lists drugs with no accepted therapeutic value and defines those people who are licensed to supply, administer and possess them. It includes cannabis, ecstasy, lysergic acid diethylamine (LSD) and mescaline.
- *Schedules 2 and 3* – these list over 100 drugs that may be administered and supplied by doctors, dentists, veterinarians and nurse prescribers to patients who may then legally possess them. A nurse may also supply these drugs but only under the directions of a doctor or dentist. A midwife can possess and administer pethidine under these schedules but only in the patient's home. A patient can only obtain the prescription from one doctor or dentist and it must be for his own use. The majority of these drugs are not in common use and those that are used are labelled 'CD' in the British National Formulary. Schedule 2 drugs include methadone, morphine, cocaine and amphetamines. Schedule 3 drugs are less potent and include pentazocine and buprenorphine. These schedules also specify how a prescription for a controlled drug should be written (see above).
- *Schedule 4* – this lists most of the benzodiazepines.
- *Schedule 5* – this exempts certain preparations containing small amounts of controlled drugs from rigid control. There is no prohibition of import, export, possession or supply of such drugs. Examples include codeine and pholcodine linctus & codeine plusphate tablets. Dihydrocodeine tablets are exempt but codeine injection is not.

The Act also defines the layout and entry-keeping of the registers that must be kept for drugs in Schedules 1 and 2.

MISUSE OF DRUGS (NOTIFICATION AND SUPPLY TO ADDICTS) REGULATIONS 1973

These were amended in 1983 and state that any doctor who has reasonable grounds to suspect that his patient is addicted to one of more of the drugs shown below must inform the Chief Medical Officer in writing within 7 days of attendance. He must supply the name, date of birth, address and NHS number of the patient wherever possible, with the date of attendance and the drug of addiction.

Drugs of addiction

- Cocaine
- Diamorphine (heroin)
- Dipipanone (Diconal)
- Methadone
- Morphine
- Opium
- Pethidine

HANDLING ILLEGAL DRUGS

You are not required by law to remove suspicious packages from patients and if you do remove illegal drugs then return them, either to the patient or a relative, then you are supplying drugs and you could be *liable to prosecution*. Such drugs should be either handed to a policeman or destroyed, although if you do destroy the drugs then you could be charged with obstruction if the police are involved. Note that if it is a Schedule 1 drug and you remove it, then you are committing an offence simply by possessing it. If you are forced to handle illicit drugs (e.g. the patient is unconscious), ensure that all your actions are witnessed and that you make witnessed contemporaneous notes. If the patient has a legally prescribed controlled drug such as methadone, then the nurse or doctor can store the drug in the controlled drugs cupboard. It can then be either administered or restored to the patient on discharge.

Patients may also transport drugs in various body cavities ('body packers' or 'mules') or swallow drugs when arrested ('body stuffers' or 'swallowers'). A doctor may then be asked to remove the drugs. In a conscious patient, this can only be done with informed consent and the patient must be made fully aware of the possible consequences of massive drug ingestion. If the patient is not able to give consent, then the doctor must act in the 'best interests' of the patient.

Note

Treat every suspicious package as if it was a bomb!

References

1. Department of Health. Drug misuse and dependence – Guidelines on Clinical Management. London: DoH, 1999
2. Brooke D, Edwards G, Andrews T. Doctors and substance misuse: types of doctor, types of problem. Addiction 1993; 88: 655–663

Further reading

British National Formulary. London: British Medical Association and the Royal Pharmaceutical Society of Great Britain

Medicines, ethics and practice: a guide for pharmacists. London: Royal Pharmaceutical Society of Great Britain

Nurse Prescribers' Formulary. London: British Medical Association/Royal Pharmaceutical Society of Great Britain/ Community Practitioners' & Health Visitors' Association/Royal College of Nursing

Glossary

Absolute privilege complete immunity from an action for libel or slander even if what was said was motivated by malice

Actual bodily harm (ABH) intentional assault occasioning physical injury

Actus reus the act of commission of a criminal offence

Admiralty law applies to British and foreign vessels and involves mostly civil matters

Advance Directive a statement made by a mentally competent adult that gives instructions about how he would wish to be treated in the event of any future loss of mental capacity

Alternative dispute resolution an alternative to civil litigation, where a third party acts as a mediator but his decision is not binding and the disputing parties must negotiate their own settlement

Arbitration an adjudication process that operates outside court, where a third party reviews the case and makes a decision that is binding on both parties

Balance of probabilities the account most likely to be the true version of events

Battery infliction of personal violence

'Best interests' decisions choices made on the behalf of incompetent patients to provide the most beneficial treatment

Body packers ('mules') people who transport drugs in various body cavities

Body stuffers ('swallowers') people who swallow drugs when arrested

Bolam standard a healthcare professional must act in accordance with a responsible and competent body of relevant professional opinion if he is not to be found negligent

Brain stem death the point at which mechanical life support should be discontinued

Caldicott guardian a member of staff (usually the Medical Director) appointed by each NHS Trust to oversee issues of confidentiality

Causation the link between actionable harm and the breach of duty of care

Child destruction the killing of a foetus in utero after 28 weeks

Civil law a private matter; proceedings are usually instituted by the injured party

Common assault threatening behaviour

Common law case or judge-made law

Concealment of birth the hiding of a body to conceal the fact of birth

Consent (implied, express) (i) *implied* – behavioural, e.g. a patient voluntarily undresses for examination; (ii) *express* – the patient gives permission orally or in writing

Contributory negligence actions of a claimant that make or made the alleged injury worse

Criminal law relates to a crime that directly and seriously threatens the well-being of the general population

Date of knowledge date on which alleged negligence occurred or when the patient became aware of the effects

Death (definition of) irreversible loss of the capacity for consciousness, combined with irreversible loss of the capacity to breathe

Death certificate (stillbirth, neonatal, cause of death) (i) *stillbirth* – after 24 weeks' gestation; (ii) *neonatal* – any death up to 28 days of age; (iii) *Medical Certificate of Cause of Death* – all other deaths

Dependence syndrome compulsion to use drugs with an over-riding focus on drug-seeking behaviour plus one or more of the following:
- Tolerance – the amount of drug needed to give the desired effect rises
- Withdrawal – both physical and psychological symptoms on stopping use
- Use of drug to relieve or avoid withdrawal symptoms

Discovery the point where all parties must produce all documents in their possession relevant to an issue in litigation

Dismissal (with notice, action short of dismissal, summary dismissal, constructive) (i) *dismissal with notice* is used for serious offences where the safety of patients is not at risk; (ii) *action short of dismissal* is used for less serious offences and includes transfer to other work or to a different location or up to 4 weeks of unpaid leave; (iii) *summary dismissal* is immediate dismissal without notice and is used for very serious offences where the welfare of the patients has been put in jeopardy; (iv) *constructive dismissal* is behaviour of an employer such that the employee is entitled to terminate his employment and consider himself dismissed

Doctrine of 'double-effect' the healthcare professional can foresee that the consequences of his actions are likely to be beneficial to the patient but could also be detrimental

Doctrine of necessity medical treatment of an unconscious patient in the absence of consent in the 'best interests' of the patient

Ecclesiastical law concerned with regulation of church affairs

Euthanasia active intervention to end life

Evidence (direct, circumstantial, hearsay) (i) *direct evidence* requires no mental processing by the judge or jury; (ii) *circumstantial evidence* requires the judge or jury to draw inferences; (iii) *hearsay evidence* is reported speech

Examination-in-chief the first line of questioning faced by a witness in court

Frozen awareness either incapable or fearful of displaying any emotion

'Gardening leave' leave on full pay for a period not usually exceeding 6 months to allow recovery from illness

Gillick competent a minor of any age considered to have sufficient understanding and intelligence to give or refuse consent

Grievous bodily harm (GBH) intentional wounding resulting in a breach in the skin

Industrial law relates to conditions of employment, trade unions and industrial relations

Infanticide the deliberate killing of an infant under the age of 12 months

Intimate body search physical examination of the orifices (ears, nostrils, mouth, rectum and vagina)

Intoximeter machine used to measure the concentration of alcohol in a breath sample

Letter of administration allows the personal representatives of a person who died intestate to give consent of the behalf of the deceased

Letter of Claim gives the dates of alleged negligent treatment and the events giving rise to the claim

Letter of Response reply to Letter of Claim, commenting on the events if they are disputed, with details of any other documentation upon which the defendant intends to rely

Living will see Advance Directive

Medicinal purpose relates to drugs used in the diagnosis, treatment or prevention of disease, induction of anaesthesia, contraception or any other permanent or temporary effect on physiological function

Medicines (POMs, P, GSL, unlicensed) (i) *prescription-only medicines (POMs)* are those that may only be supplied or administered on the instruction of a doctor, dentist or nurse prescriber; (ii) *pharmacy-only medicines (P)* are those that may only be bought from a registered pharmacy, under the supervision of a pharmacist; (iii) *general sale list medicines (GSLs)* are those that can be bought from any retail outlet; (iv) *unlicensed medicines* are those with no product licence and no manufacturer liability

Mens rea the intention to commit a criminal offence

Mental disorder mental illness, arrested or incomplete development of mind, psychopathic disorder or any other disorder or disability of mind

Mental impairment a state of arrested or incomplete development of mind which includes significant impairment of intelligence and social functioning and is associated with abnormally aggressive or seriously irresponsible conduct on the part of the person concerned

Newton hearing occurs when the accused pleads guilty and the judge elects to hear from the prosecution and defence in order to decide sentencing

Orders of court – children (contact, prohibited steps, residence, specific issues) (i) *contact order*

defines persons with whom the child must be allowed to have contact; (ii) *prohibited steps order* stops a person with parental responsibility from making certain decisions over the child's welfare without recourse to the courts; (iii) *residence order* defines where and with whom the child will live; (iv) *specific issues order* gives directions for dealing with a particular aspect of the child's care

Patient group directions the supply and administration of a named medicine or vaccine in a known clinical situation where patients may not be identified prior to arrival

Permanent vegetative state the brain stem still functions but the cortex does not; the patient can breathe unaided and the autonomic nervous system works but he cannot see, hear, speak, feel pain or move voluntarily

Personal misconduct inappropriate behaviour unrelated to clinical skills

Physician-assisted suicide a doctor prescribes a lethal drug but it is either administered by the patient or by a third party

Polymerase chain reaction (PCR) new, more accurate method of DNA profiling using minute quantities of material; chance of a random match < 1 in several million

Professional incompetence inadequate or poor performance of clinical skills or judgement

Professional misconduct inappropriate behaviour arising during the exercise of clinical skills

'Proofing' the defendant's solicitors prepare answers to the particulars of the claim

Protected disclosure disclosure of confidential information concerning matters of public interest to only the relevant bodies

Psychopathic disorder a persistent disorder or disability of mind (whether or not including significant impairment of intelligence) that results in abnormally aggressive or seriously irresponsible conduct on the part of the person concerned

Quantifiable harm disability, loss or injury suffered as a result of negligence by another

Quantum the amount of financial compensation for the harm suffered as a result of negligence by another

Risk management the ability to detect, analyse and learn from adverse events

Service law applies to all serving members of the Navy, Air Force and Army; administered through courts martial

Severe mental impairment a state of arrested or incomplete development of mind that includes severe impairment of intelligence and social functioning and is associated with abnormally aggressive or seriously irresponsible conduct on the part of the person concerned

Shaken baby syndrome a clinical and pathological entity characterized by retinal and subdural and/or subarachnoid haemorrhages with minimal or absent signs of external trauma

Statute law   law that is enacted by Parliament

Subpoena   a writ calling a person to attend at court

'Substitutive judgement' decisions   the decision maker must provide the treatment that the patient would have chosen had he still been competent; tend to be based on quality, rather than quantity of life

'Three wise men' procedure   used to deal with incapacity in healthcare professionals due to physical or mental disability, including addiction

Tin ear   bruising of the pinna of the ear caused by slap to the side of the head

Tolerance   physiological changes within the body so that larger amounts of alcohol or drugs of addiction must be consumed in order to achieve the same effects

Tort   a civil wrong, dealt with through civil proceedings

Tutor-dative   a person appointed under the *Adults with Incapacity (Scotland) Act 2000* who has the authority to make medical decisions on behalf of an incompetent patient

Vicarious liability   legal responsibility for the actions of juniors or other staff

Withdrawal (from drug dependence)   both physical and psychological symptoms if the drug is not taken

Withdrawal/withholding of treatment   treatment is either stopped or not started on the basis that it would be of no benefit to the patient

Witness (of fact, professional, expert)   (i) *witness of fact* is one who gives factual evidence; (ii) a *professional witness* is one who also provides factual evidence but can give some opinions; (iii) an *expert witness* is one who provides both fact and opinion evidence and guides the court over matters that are the subject of special expertise

Xenotransplantation   the transfer of viable cells, tissues or organs between species

Yellow Card scheme   method by which healthcare professionals can report any adverse drug reactions to the Committee on Safety of Medicines

Appendix

Legislation covering legal aspects of medicine

Chapter	Subject	Related legislation (UK unless stated otherwise)
1	Criminal law	*Prosecution of Offenders Act 1985*
	Statute interpretation	*Interpretation Act 1978*
	District judges	*Access to Justice Act 1999*
	Youth Court	*Criminal Justice Act 1991*
	Crown Court	*Courts Act 1971*
2	Crown Prosecution Service	*Prosecution of Offenders Act 1995*
	Arrest and prosecution	*Police and Criminal Evidence Act (PACE) 1984*
	Disclosure of evidence	*Criminal Procedure and Investigations act 1996*
		Criminal Procedure (Scotland) Act 1995
	Expert witness role	Civil Procedure Rules 1998
3	Statements in criminal cases	*Criminal Justice Act 1967* (Section 9)
		Magistrates Courts Act 1980 (Section 102)
		Magistrates Courts Rules 1981 (Rule 90)
	Statement on behalf of someone else	*Criminal Justice Act 1988* (documentary hearsay)
4	Forensic samples (collection)	*Police and Criminal Evidence Act (PACE) 1984*
		Prisoners and Criminal Proceedings (Scotland) Act 1993
		Road Traffic Act 1988
	Intimate searches	*Misuse of Drugs Act 1971*
		Police and Criminal Evidence Act (PACE) 1984
5	Consent to procedure	*Human Fertilisation and Embryology Act 1990*

Chapter	Subject	Related legislation (UK unless stated otherwise)
	Tutor-dative	*Adults with Incapacity (Scotland) Act 2000*
	Consent and minors	*Age of Legal Capacity (Scotland) Act 1991*
		Age of Minority Act 1969 (Northern Ireland)
		Children (Scotland) Act 1995
		Children Act 1989
		Family Law Reform Act 1969 (England & Wales)
	Consent in special cases	*Children and Young Persons Act 1933*
	Consent – incompetent patient	*Human Rights Act 1998*
		Mental Health Act 1983
6	Confidentiality	*Human Rights Act 1998*
	Disclosure:	
	– public interest	*Ontario Medicine Act 1991*
		Police Act 1964
		Public Interest Disclosure Act 1998
	– data protection	*Access to Health Records Act 1990* (England, Wales, Scotland)
		Access to Health Records Act 1994 (Northern Ireland)
		Consumer Protection Act 1987
		Data Protection Act 1998
	– employers/insurers	*Access to Medical Reports Act 1988* (England, Wales, Scotland)
		Access to Personal Files and Medical Reports (NI) Order 1991 (Northern Ireland)
	– teaching/audit/research	*Data Protection Act 1998*
	– adverse drug reactions	*Data Protection Act 1998*
	– civil litigation	*Data Protection Act 1998*
		Supreme Court Act 1981
	– criminal proceedings	*Criminal Procedure (Scotland) Act 1995*
		Criminal Procedure and Investigations Act 1996
		Police and Criminal Evidence Act (PACE) 1984

Chapter	Subject	Related legislation (UK unless stated otherwise)
	Breach of confidentiality – controlled circumstances	*Prevention of Terrorism (Temporary Provisions) Act 2000* *Abortion Act 1991* *AIDS (Control) Act 1987* *Births and Deaths Registration Act 1953* *Control of Substances Hazardous to Health (COSHH) Regulations* *Factories Act 1895* *Human Fertilisation and Embryology (Disclosure of Information) Act 1992* *Human Fertilisation and Embryology Act 1990* *Misuse of Drugs (Notification and Supply to Addicts) Regulations 1985* *Misuse of Drugs Act 1971* *NHS (Notification of Births and Deaths) Regulations 1982* *NHS (Venereal Disease) Regulations 1974* *Perjury Act 1911* *Prevention of Terrorism (Temporary Provisions) Act 2000* *Public Health (Control of Disease) Act 1984* *Public Health (Infectious Diseases) Regulations 1988* *Road Traffic Act 1988*
7	Risk management Clinical negligence	*Health and Safety at Work Act 1974* *NHS and Community Care Act 1990 (Section 21)*
8	Health Service Ombudsman	*Health Service Commissioners Act 1993*
9	Contributory negligence Negligence claim – time limitation	*Social Security Administration Act 1992* (England, Wales, Scotland) *Social Security Administration (Northern Ireland) Act 1992* *Vaccine Damage Payments Act 1979* *Limitation Act 1980*

Chapter	Subject	Related legislation (UK unless stated otherwise)
10	General Medical Council:	
	– establishment	*Medical Act 1858*
	– powers, including discipline	*Medical Act 1983*
	– education	*European Specialist Medical Qualifications Order 1995*
	Committee on Professional Performance	*Medical (Professional Performance) Act 1995*
	UKCC (NMC)	*Health Act 1983*
		Nurses, Midwives and Health Visitors Act 1979
		Nurses, Midwives and Health Visitors Act 1992
		Nursing and Midwifery Order 2001
	Professions supplementary to medicine	*Professions Supplementary to Medicine Act 1960*
	NHS tribunal	*NHS Act 1977*
		Tribunals and Inquiries Act 1992
	Protected disclosure	*Public Interest Disclosure Act 1998*
11	Death certification	*Births and Deaths Registration Act 1953* (England & Wales)
		Coroner's Act (Northern Ireland) 1959
		Fatal Accidents and Sudden Deaths Inquiry (Scotland) Act 1976
		Registration of Births, Deaths and Marriages (Scotland) Act 1965
	Coroner system	*Coroners Act 1988*
	Post mortem/removal of tissue	*Human Tissue Act 1961*
		Human Tissue Act 1962 (Northern Ireland)
	Disposal	*Anatomy Act 1984*
		Births and Deaths Registration Act 1926
12	Organ donation, organ retrieval	*Human Tissue Act 1961*
		Human Tissue Act 1962 (Northern Ireland)
	Payment for organs	*Human Organ Transplants Act 1989*
	Living donor	*Human Organ Transplants Act 1989*
		Human Organ Transplants (Unrelated Persons) Regulations 1989

Chapter	Subject	Related legislation (UK unless stated otherwise)
13	Physician-assisted suicide	*Burial and Cremation Act 1991* (Holland)
		Death with Dignity Act 1994 (USA)
		Rights of the Terminally Ill Act 1996 (Australia, Northern Territory)
		Termination of Life on Request and Assisted Suicide Review Act 2002 (Holland)
	Advance Directive	*Adults with Incapacity (Scotland) Act 2000*
		Children Act 1989
		Mental Health Act 1983
		Natural Death Act of California 1976 (USA, California)
		Patient Self-Determination Act 1991 (USA)
14	Infanticide	*Infanticide Act 1938*
	Stillbirth	*Stillbirth (Definition) Act 1992*
		Still-Births (Scotland) Act 1938
	Child destruction	*Infant Life Preservation Act 1929*
	Concealment of birth	*Concealment of Birth (Scotland) Act 1809*
		Offences against the Person Act 1861 (England & Wales)
	Children Acts	*Children Act 1989* (England & Wales)
		Children (Scotland) Act 1995
15	Mental health	*Mental Health Act 1983*
		Mental Health Act 1984 (Scotland)
16	Drink driving	*Road Traffic Act 1988*
17	Drugs	
	– prescribing	*Medicinal Products: Prescription by Nurses Act 1992*
	– misuse	*Dangerous Drugs Acts –1965, 1967*
		Drugs (Prevention of Misuse) Act 1964
		Misuse of Drugs (Notification and Supply to Addicts) Regulations 1973
		Misuse of Drugs (Safe Custody) Regulations 1973
		Misuse of Drugs Act 1971 (England, Wales, Scotland)
		Misuse of Drugs Regulations 1985
	Safety of medicines	*Medicines Act 1968*

Index

Temperature, body
  coma due to hypothermia, 148
  time of death and, 134–5
Termination of Life on Request and Assisted Suicide (Review) Act (Holland 2002), 161
Terrorism, disclosure, 74, 76
Thalidomide disaster, 220
Thermal injuries, *see* Burns; Scalds
Third tier courts, 8
'Three wise men' procedure, 124
  definition, 124, 229
Tin ear, 177, 229
Tissues, *see* Organs
Tolerance (drug), 219, 229
Tort
  definition, 229
  law of, 2
Toxicological evidence, *Road Traffic Act (1988)*, 209–10
Transfusions and Jehovah's witnesses, 55
Transplantation, organ/tissue
  donation, 152–6
    authorisation for removal, 153–4
    donor management, 152–4
    legislation, 153, 154, 155, 156, 234
    removal and storage, 154
    supply and demand for organs, 155–6
  non-human sources, *see* Xenotransplantation
Treasure trove, 142
Treatment
  consent, *see* Consent
  description of any, in police statement, 31
  disclosure of risk, 51–2
  instructions about wish for, after future loss of mental capacity, *see* Advance Directives
  Mental Health Act and
    admission for treatment, 192, 195, 200
    consent and second opinion, 198
    Scotland, 200
    urgent treatment, 198, 200
  refusal, *see* Advance Directives
  withdrawal and withholding, 162–3
    definition, 229
    principles, 162–3
Trials (clinical), consent, 57, *see also* Research

Trials (court), mode, 7, 18–19
Tribunals and Inquiries Act (1992), 125
Trusts, *see* NHS
Tutor-dative, 53, 168, 229

U
UK, *see* United Kingdom
UKCC, Nursing and Midwifery Council replacing, 116
Ulster, *see* Northern Ireland
Unconscious patients, consent and, 52–3, *see also* Coma
Unfitness to practice proceedings, NMC, 118–19
United Kingdom Central Council, Nursing and Midwifery Council replacing, 116
United Kingdom Transplant Support Service Authority, 154
United States of America (USA)
  Advance Directives, 165
    history, 164
  euthanasia, history, 160–1
Unlicensed medicines, 221, 227
Unrelated Live Transplant Regulatory Authority (ULTRA), 156
Urine samples, 41–2, 44–6
  taken under *Road Traffic Act*, 212
USA, *see* United States of America

V
Vaginal swab, 45
Vegetative state, permanent, *see* Permanent vegetative state
Venereal diseases, confidentiality issues, 75
Ventilation, non-therapeutic, illegality, 152
Verbal (oral) warning in hospital disciplinary procedure, 121
Verdicts, 20
  Coroner's, 142
Vestibulo-ocular reflex, 151
Vicarious liability, 102, 229
Viscera, *see* Organs
Visual impairment and driving, 213
Volatile substance abuse, 219
Voluntary Euthanasia Society, Advance Directives and, 164
Vulval swab, 45